Navy SEAL Exercises

Cutting Edge Fitness
Total Body Workout

Mark De Lisle
United States Navy SEAL

COPYRIGHT

Author: Mark De Lisle
United States Navy SEAL

LIBRARY OF CONGRESS

Catalogueing-in-Publication Data

DE LISLE, Mark
    Navy SEAL Exercises: Cutting Edge Total Body Workout

    1.   Physical Fitness.
        United States Navy SEAL Physical Fitness Training Program.
        Total Body Workout Levels: Beginner, Intermediate, Advanced.
        Personal Progress Record and Charts.   Nutrition Guides.
        Anatomic Illustrations.

        ISBN   0-9654093-0-9

FIRST EDITION

PUBLISHER

Cutting Edge Fitness
4901 Morena Boulevard, Suite 127
San Diego, CA 92117 USA

(800) 281-SEAL (281-7325)

PRODUCTION

Publication Edited, Designed, Typography, Illustrations [© Anatomical Drawings, © Cartoons, Logos], and Navy SEAL Training Program Photography by:

Cheryl Ann Allison
Post Office Box 182302
Coronado, CA 92178 USA

Front Cover and Exterior Training Photography:
Victor Sotelo

PRINTED IN THE UNITED STATES OF AMERICA

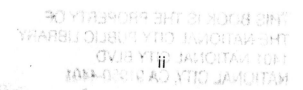

Training Advisement

Resolve to stop thinking negative thoughts, such as "I can't—there's too much for me to overcome," and start saying "I *can!* I *will!* *Nobody* will stop me!" Each day is a new day and a new start—so make yours with Cutting Edge Fitness.

Do not be fooled by the simplicity of these exercises. Anybody can flip through this book, like flipping through a picture magazine, and say "This is it?" The key to this program is the format in which the exercises are performed, i.e., the pyramid system, and the complete *blitzing* of all muscle groups that cause its effectiveness. If you are not sore after starting this program, or in better terms—if your muscles are not "burning" from exertion, you did not use the system properly.

— Mark De Lisle

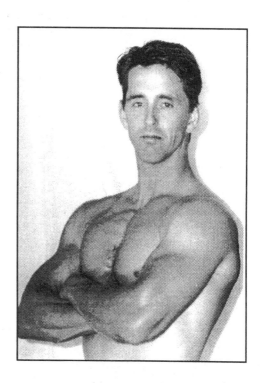

Disclaimer

CONSULT A PHYSICIAN before you begin this or any strenuous exercise program or diet modification, especially if you have [or suspect you may have] heart disease, high blood pressure, diabetes, or any other adverse medical condition.

WARNING: If you feel faint or dizzy at any time while performing any portion of this training program, stop immediately and seek medical evaluation.

The author and publisher disclaim any liability, personal or professional, resulting from the misapplication of any training procedure described in this publication.

Dedication

This book is dedicated to all UDT/SEALs, past and present, who have perfected the meaning of perserverance and commitment.

And with special thanks to my family and Cristina Uribe, who have been the inspiration behind this book with their love and support the entire way.

I also extend my gratitude to R. J. Wolf, without whose efforts this endeavor would not be possible.

— Mark De Lisle

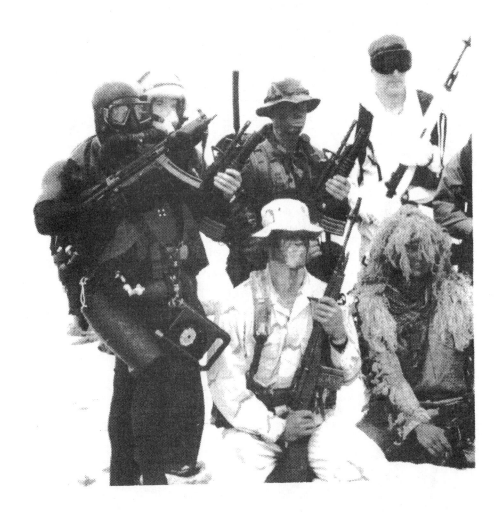

Contents

U. S. Navy SEAL Training Program   12

Contents

Introduction

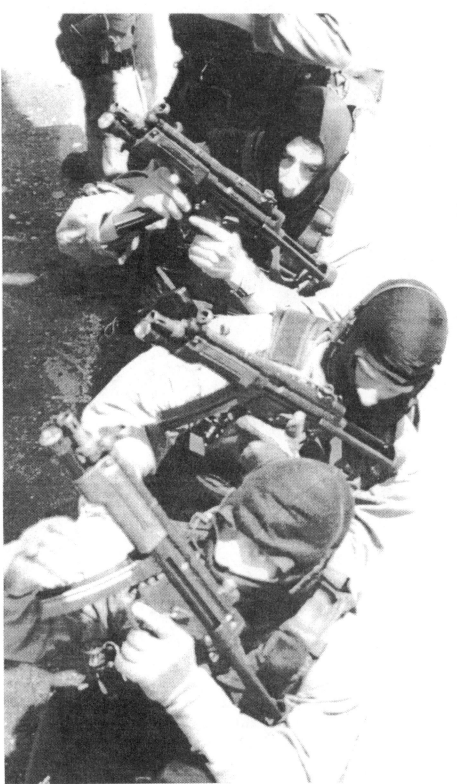

Throughout the past decade the public has become increasingly aware of an elite group of men known as Navy SEALs.

Without soliciting publicity, Navy SEALs have become recognized as some of the fittest men in all the world.

Today, SEALs can be seen in anything from *Muscle and Fitness* magazine to the Discovery channel on cable television.

This training program will help explain how these unique and dedicated men have achieved world prominence and an extraordinary reputation for physical fitness.

SEAL History & Training

SEAL History

My purpose here is not to give you a complete and in-depth review of SEAL history, rather, a basic understanding of who we are and where we came from. Also, you will better understand why it is paramount for us to excel in all areas of physical fitness and mental development.

In the early 1960s President John F. Kennedy, envisioning the path modern warfare was heading, decided to organize an elite group of men specializing in counter-terrorist tactics. SEALs (the acronym for Sea, Air and Land) were taken from the ranks of the United States Navy Underwater Demolition Teams [UDT].

All SEALs get their roots from the "frogmen" of World War II, who successfully performed covert amphibious missions against incredible odds. During the 1960s "frogmen" began forming into what is known today as Navy SEALs. By 1983 the term "UDT" was eliminated, and all UDT teams became SEAL teams.

Vietnam was the first arena for Navy SEALs to be showcased and prove their value as a combat unit. They proved themselves ten-fold, leaving Vietnam as the highest decorated unit and with the highest kill-per-person ratio of any U.S. combat unit. SEALs were so feared by the Viet Cong, they were called "devils with green faces!"

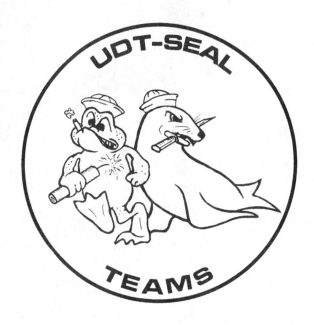

SEAL Training

SEALs come from all walks of life—but that does not mean *anyone* can be a Navy SEAL. You have to earn the right of passage.

This is where BUD/S comes into the picture. BUD/S stands for Basic Underwater Demolition/SEAL School, located in Coronado, California, USA. This is where all initial training for SEAL candidates are held. All candidates—officers and enlisted men alike—are required to pass the same tests. The training is excruciating and bordering on impossible.

BUD/S is broken into four phases. Upon arrival, you begin Fourth Phase. This is the preparatory phase, and the only phase where instructors can show a little bit of their human side. You begin running, swimming, and performing difficult exercises, improving your techniques daily. After an average of two months you take an entrance physical test to determine if you are ready to make the next class for First Phase.

Once the First Phase class is finalized, there is a traditional party on the beach the Saturday night before class begins. This is where all SEAL candidates shave their heads and celebrate wildly, because as of Monday—*life ends as you know it.* You are now property of the SEAL instructors.

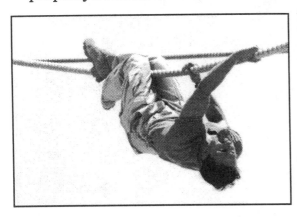

First Phase is very demanding. The sixth week of First Phase is the infamous "Hell Week!" I'll explain more about that later.[1] After "Hell Week" we were given one week in tennis shoes to allow the swelling in our feet to go down. Soon we were back in jungle boots. Now we were qualified to learn SEAL tactics, stealth, concealment, and Hydro Reconnaissance.

Then came Second Phase, or Dive Phase. Here we learned about scuba diving with open air scuba tanks. Once we gained the instructors' confidence, we were allowed to use pure oxygen tanks.

The stamina required for such grueling training was taking its toll, and the numbers in our class continued to dwindle. We started out with a class of 130, and at this phase of training we were down to 75.

The last and final phase, Land Warfare, was spent half in Coronado and half on San Clemente Island. We learned everything from land navigation and demolition tactics to small firearms.

We also had to increase our speed and endurance because the qualifying times for running and swimming were getting shorter and shorter. Even though our bodies were falling apart from the grueling training, we managed to keep up and pass the tests.

I'll never forget the feeling coming back from San Clemente Island, knowing I only had one more week of training left—walking tall and proud!

---

1. "Hell Week" is described on page 6.

My Story

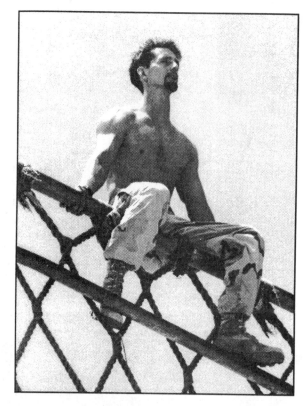

Having just gone through a divorce, I needed to get my head on straight and get some stability back into my life. I wanted to finish my college degree in marketing, but I was not in a financial position to cover the cost of college. Taking my father's recommendation I entered the Navy, hoping to utilize their college programs and complete my degree.

While at boot camp in San Diego, California a recruiter came in and showed us a film about the SEAL program titled "Be Someone Special." My eyes lit up when I saw the training and skills required of a modern-day SEAL. I immediately knew that this was for me. Never one to sit behind a desk from nine to five, I just had to find out—to be pushed to my absolute limit. I kept asking myself if I could make it. My body was nearing 27 years, and I had been out of shape since my football days in college six years ago. *Could I do it?*

"Many people close to me doubted I could achieve my goal, but I refused to let anyone stop me ... "

I took the entrance exam and barely passed. Now I was really excited. I was going to get the electronic training I wanted, and also have the chance to become a Navy SEAL. Then, two weeks before graduation from boot camp, a counselor called me in and informed me that the electronics class was full, and that I would not be able to attend. Instead, I was offered three other classifications and I chose Quartermaster.

After graduating from boot camp as the top recruit, I was off to Orlando, Florida, for Quartermaster training.

Once there, I was informed I had to take the extrance exam to BUD/S (SEAL School) all over again! I was caught off guard and as it turned out—this policy was only for Orlando! I was worried and started to panic because I had already lost the opportunity for electronic training, and I didn't want to lose SEAL training as well. My entire career suddenly came down to one test that never should have been required. Have you ever been in that position?

Although I stayed in good shape since boot camp, my pull-ups were lacking. Sure enough, the day of the test I passed everything—except the pull-ups. While doing the last pull-up, the instructor told me to do just *one more* because I jerked my foot too much.

"There were many times I didn't know if I would make it through a test or evaluation, but each time I dug deep inside myself and found strength and determination I didn't know I possessed."

It all came down to one last pull-up for me to qualify for SEAL training. *And I just couldn't do it!* I had nothing left in me, and my chin would not make it over the bar. I hopped off the bar in disbelief. My worse nightmare came true—and my dreams were shattered. Then I became furious and told myself, "Mark, get off your rear and start working on your pull-ups. You will not let them beat you. You will not quit!" I had enough time for one more test before graduation from Quartermaster School. *Nothing* was going to stop me from passing the test this time!

Finally, Judgment Day came! I passed the beginning portion of the test—and then it was time for pull-ups. Something sparked in me and I performed pull-up after pull-up without a problem. I did three more than required. I wanted to prove to the instructor that I had what it takes to become a SEAL, and erase any doubt in their minds. I hopped off the bar and was silent, then it hit me—I'm going to BUD/S! I soon graduated from the Orlando school in the top 5% of my class and was off to San Diego, California for SEAL training.

In March, 1991 I arrived at BUD/S and to my surprise, it felt as though it were summer. I was immediately in love with San Diego, California. There are beautiful beaches everywhere, and the suburb of Coronado, where SEAL training is held, is like something straight out of a movie. Many views throughout the city are breathtaking.

After I checked into BUD/S and received my basic gear, I began training in Fourth Phase. Every phase of BUD/S has its own unique tests and obstacles to overcome.

The Infamous "Hell Week"

Only the best survive at BUD/S. You have to stay extremely alert and focused, while never letting your guard down. The best example of this is "Hell Week." This is the week that all BUD/S students must pass somehow— *some way* —if they want to become a Navy SEAL. During this week, every training scenario you have learned up to that point is executed. There were many times I didn't know if I would make it through a test or evaluation, but each time I dug deep inside myself and found strength and determination I didn't know I possessed.

Throughout the entire week you only get a half hour of sleep, here and there, and never more than two hours total for the week. The majority of time you are soaking wet—either from hoses or "surf torture." Surf torture is where you have to get in the ocean's surf zone and let the waves crash down on your face. The extensive amount of time we had to spend in the surf zone brought us dangerously close to hypothermia, and many SEAL candidates were disqualified during this exercise. Somehow, I made it through Hell Week—taking one day at a time—and not looking too far into the future.

> *"Throughout the entire week you only get a half hour of sleep, here and there, and never more than two hours total for the week."*

Once through Hell Week and First Phase, I was ready for Dive Phase (Second Phase) and Land Warfare (Third Phase). After completing both, an unbelievable dream came true—BUD/S graduation! I finished, phase by phase, and created new friends and bonds that will last a lifetime.

It was a very emotional time for me, and I was very proud of myself. Many people close to me doubted I could achieve my goal, but I refused to let anyone stop me. I was 28 years old, in the best shape of my life, faster and stronger than when I was 18—and just accomplished what guys 6 to 8 years younger than me had done.

My next assignment was SEAL Team Three—and the dream continued!

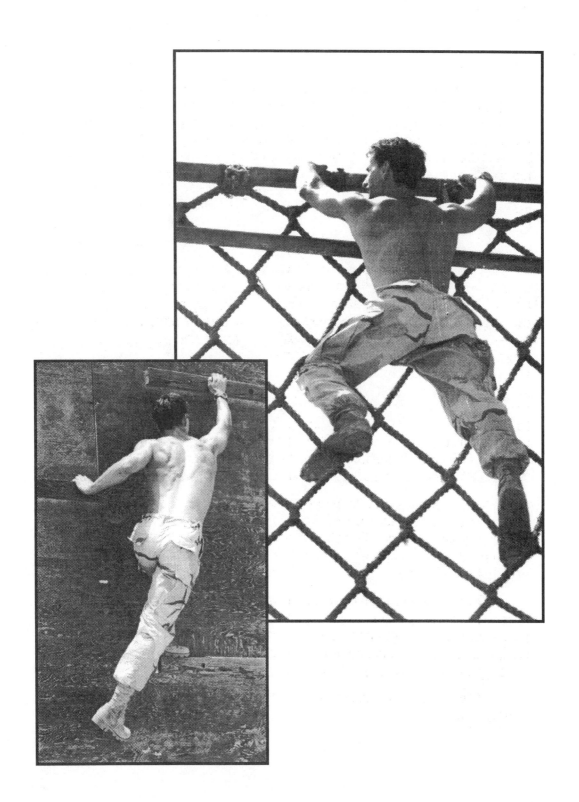

You Can Do It!

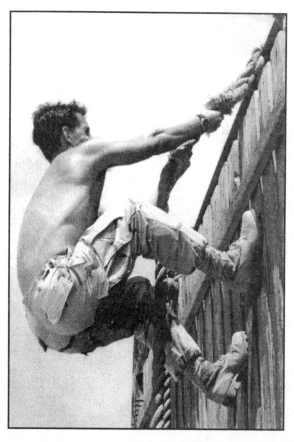

Many people believe the only way to get in shape is by putting a lot of money into trendy fitness centers, or spending hard-earned cash on a variety of workout video tapes. In the end, these methods seldom give us the results we are looking for. But don't get me wrong—I am not demeaning the value of gyms or workout tapes, and I still enjoy the benefits of a gym to keep fit. Weight lifting and other facilities available there can be extremely beneficial. However, to obtain and maintain supreme cardiovascular fitness and a rock-hard body, I must continually use the training regiment I learned as a member of the Navy SEALs.

You will find that I use the word "results" quite often. Isn't that the key word we are looking for? This program was not developed solely to motivate you. I will not give you any false hopes. No, this program is for someone who is motivated and seeking their ultimate level of fitness! I will not guarantee 100% results. No program can truthfully guarantee 100% results because everyone has a different level of motivation and fitness. If anyone guarantees you 100% results, then you are being deceived. However, I can tell you from painful personal experience that results can only come from dedication and a deep desire within yourself.

"if you are tired of being out of shape, or perhaps seeking an incredible challenge, then use this program and watch your body reach fitness levels you never dreamed possible. I did!"

If you are tired of being out of shape, or perhaps seeking an incredible challenge—then use this program and watch your body reach fitness levels you never dreamed possible. *I did!*

As I mentioned before, there are some decent gyms out there—but no one can deny the Navy SEALs reputation in fitness is second to none. I've seen people lose 20 lbs. in one month and fitness levels skyrocket using these exact same exercises that you, too, can perform in your own backyard.

The Mental Edge

SEALs are frequently asked, "How were you able to make it through such torturous training? Were you an exceptional swimmer or runner?" The most common answer is "I was mentally tough!" In addition to superior athletic ability and physical fitness, one thing all SEALs have in common that enables them to survive training is *determination*. The central driving force of success is in your own mind, which is the key to all of your strength and motivation. If you want results from this program—then start strengthening yourself *mentally*.

The biggest impression that SEAL training has left on me is that your body will perform beyond limits you never thought possible to achieve. Never doubt this program will work for you! Thousands of SEALs, past and present, can testify that it does!

Here are some tips to help you get started.

● First, be determined to succeed !

Clearly identify the fitness results you want—and vow to yourself that no individual or obstacle is going to stop you from achieving your goal.

● Put your goals down on paper.

A goal not written is just a dream! A written goal is more than just a dream—it's a clearly defined objective.

Create long term goals and short term goals. Write down your long term goals, then set short term or smaller goals to achieve your ultimate goal. By concentrating on and accomplishing your short term goals, you will achieve your long term goals!

● Review your goals often to stay motivated.

Keep your list of goals in an area of high visibility, so you can read them often and stay motivated. With this attitude you will be ready to achieve a rock-hard body in an incredibly short amount of time.

● **Make a visual record of your progress.**

Take a picture of yourself before you start this program and every three months thereafter, so you can visually monitor your progress. You are going to be so amazed!

Determine in your mind what you want to look like and don't compromise. With this program, your goals can be reached.

Record your desired weight, measurements, and endurance level through each phase. [For your convenience, forms to record your progress are included in Section IX of this book]

● **Above all, remember this:**

I did it—and so can you!

Now get busy!

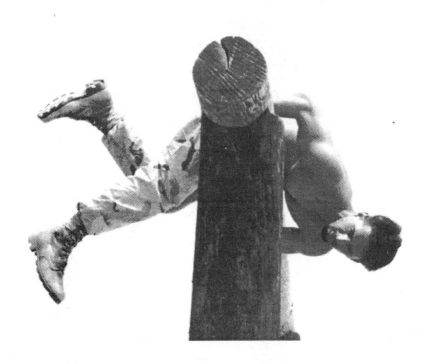

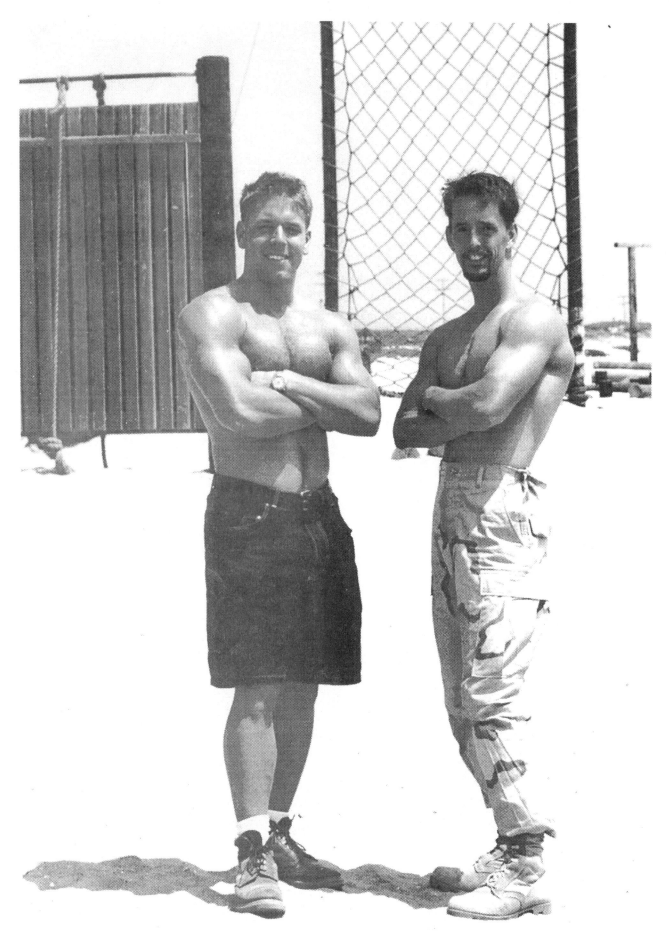

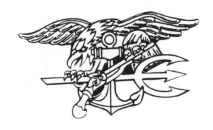

U. S. Navy SEAL
Training Program

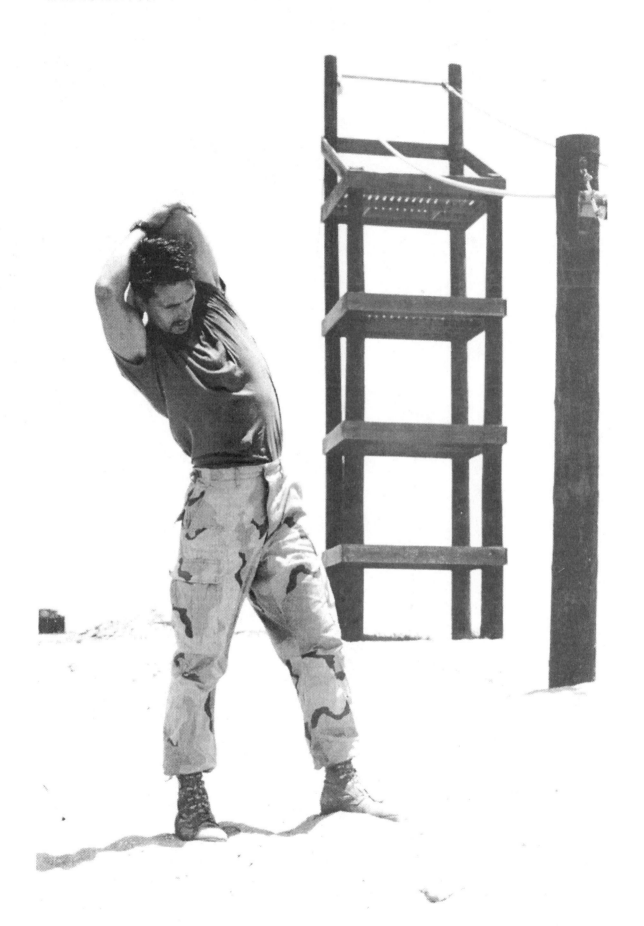

I. Stretching

I. Stretching

Stretching can be one of the most neglected areas of a workout.   I cannot stress the importance of stretching enough. As a Navy SEAL, I could not perform at the peak levels expected of me without first warming up my body.   Due to stiffness or a lack of motion, your joint structures, tendons, ligaments and muscles will easily tear.   By stretching, we allow ourselves a greater range of motion, which in turn prevents injuries.

You will achieve your best range of motion and flexibility if your muscles are lightly worked before stretching. For example, it used to be taught that the key to effective flexibility was stretching while your muscles were cold, and before any activity.   It is now known that stretching cold muscles is *not* the most efficient method.

"I can not express the importance of stretching enough. As a Navy SEAL, I could not perform at the peak levels required of me without first warming up my body."

Before actually stretching it is best to start with 2 to 5 minutes of jumping jacks and push-ups, to warm up the upper body, and/or 5 minutes of light jogging or bicycle riding, to warm the legs. This gets the blood flowing into the muscles and makes them more pliable and able to stretch, preparing them for a more effective stretching session. Once this step is finished, and only when you feel warm, begin stretching.

Throughout these stretches remember to stretch *slowly*. Try to hold each stretch for at least 15 seconds—and **never** bounce! You should feel pulling, not pain.   "Pulling" can be described as a gradual discomfort or soreness due to tight muscles. As you stretch longer, tightness will decrease and flexibility will increase. "Pain" can be described as a sharp, intense sensation causing great discomfort to a specific point. This can happen when you do not stretch slowly. As you continue your daily stretching you will be able to distinguish pulling from pain and recognize how to loosen your muscles.

Using the stretches I have listed here, your total pre-workout stretching time should be approximately 15 minutes.   When your workout is completed, do at least 10 more minutes of stretching. This is when you will be most limber and achieve the greatest gain in flexibility.   Not only is it important to stretch before and after exercising, but also during the exercise program. While you are working out your muscle fibers begin to tighten. By stretching during your workout you loosen up your muscle fibers, allowing more fibers to be affected—which allows much greater results.

A. Upper Body Stretches

1. Upper Body Stretch

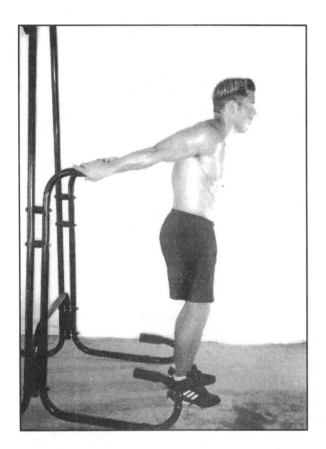

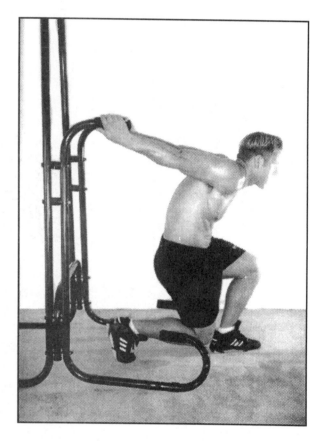

Figure 1

- Find something you can grab onto with both hands, at about chest level.

- Place both arms behind you and grab this object, palms down.

Figure 2

- Lean forward, then to the right, and then to the left.

- Lean as far as you can each way.

- Concentrate on stretching your chest and your arms.

- To get the best stretch possible, do this exercise *slowly.*

A. Upper Body Stretches

2. Single Arm Stretch

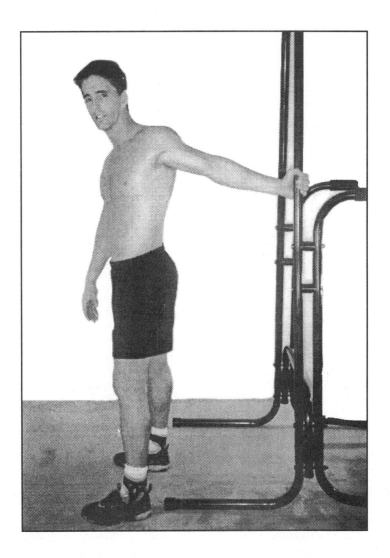

Figure 1

- Find something you can grab onto with both hands, at about chest level.

- Place one arm behind you and grab this object, palm down.

- Stretch only one arm at a time. Isolating each side increases the effectiveness of the stretch.

- Muscle flexibility will enable you to perform a greater number of repetitions. The more repetitions you perform will increase your muscle strength and development.

- To get the best stretch possible, do this exercise *slowly*.

A. Upper Body Stretches

3. Tricep Stretch

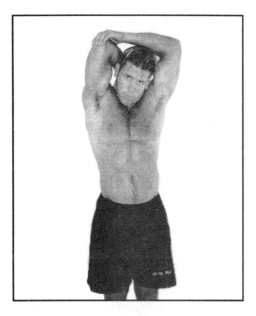

Figure 1

Place your right hand behind your head and down the middle of your back, as far as it will go.

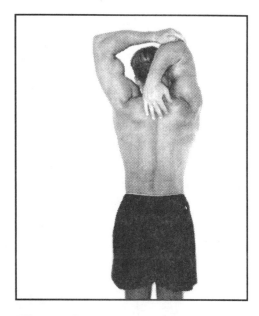

Figure 2

Now place your left hand on your right elbow and begin stretching toward your left.

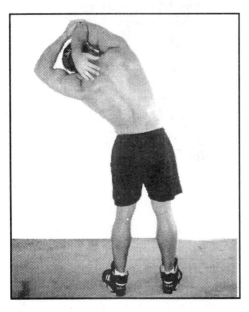

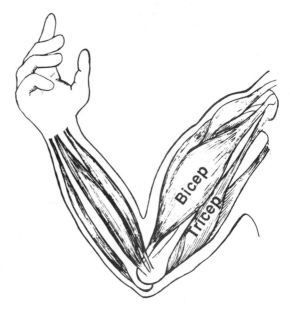

Figure 3

- Once you reach that *discomfort* zone, maintain that position for 15 to 30 seconds.

- Switch sides.

A. Upper Body Stretches

4.   Shoulder Stretch

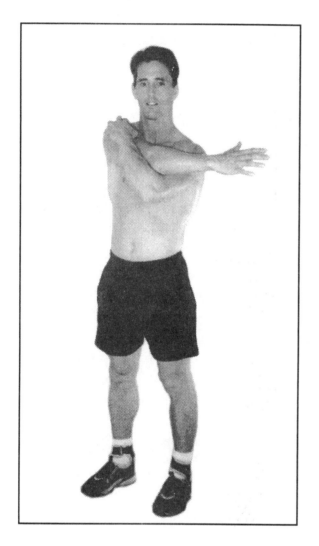

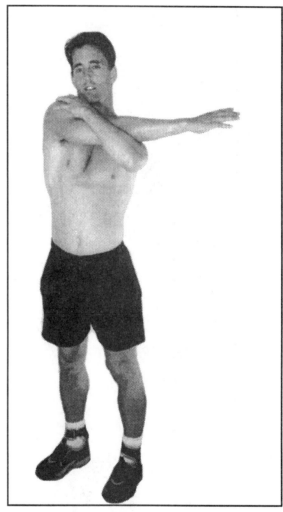

Figure 1

- Bring your right arm across your chest.

- Place your right elbow in the inside joint of your left arm, then reach across and grab your right shoulder.

Figure 2

- Squeeze and elevate your right elbow upward.

- Hold this position for 15 to 30 seconds.

- Switch sides.

A. Upper Body Stretches

5. Two-Person Chest Stretch

If you have a partner, this is an excellent stretch for the chest and biceps. Main emphasis should be on you. Arms should not be forced together.

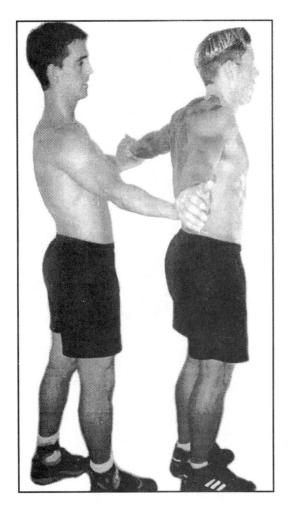

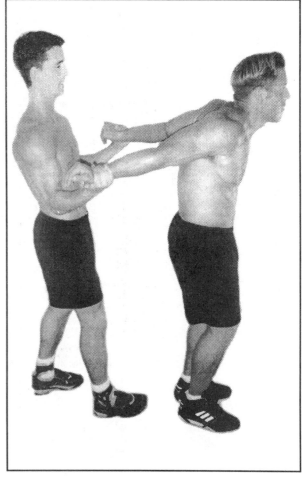

Figure 1

- Place hands behind you with thumbs up, palms facing out.

- Partner behind you places his hands on your wrists.

Figure 2

- Partner carefully brings your wrists together, as close as possible.

- Hold this position for 15 seconds, then release.

20

A. Upper Body Stretches

6.   Fore & Aft Stretch

This stretch will help stretch your abs and your lower back. To prevent added stress to the back, it is important to keep your back straight wile bending over with your knees slightly bent. This is a good stretch to perform before and after the ab routine.

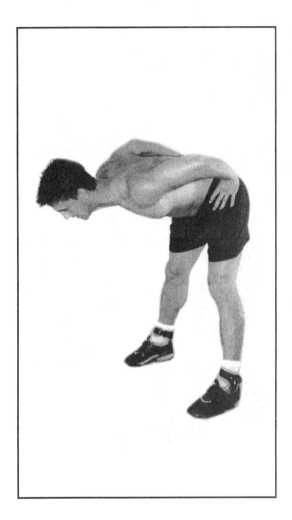

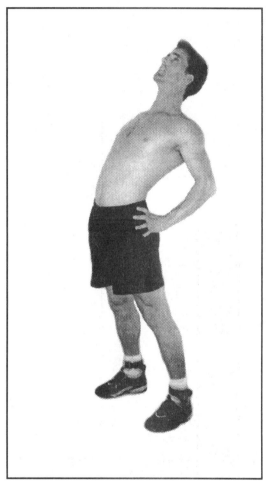

Figure 1

- Stand with legs shoulder-width apart, hands on your hips.

- Slowly bend forward, keeping your lower back straight.

- Once you have reached the point where your back begins to get tight, take a deep breath and as you exhale, try stretching a little more.

- Hold this position for 15 seconds.

Figure 2

- Now lean back, pushing your hips until your stomach is tight.

- Hold this position for 15 seconds.

A. Upper Body Stretches

7. Swimmer Stretch

This is a good stretch for the chest and anterior deltoids.
It can be used before and after the push-up segment.
*Perform stretch slowly.

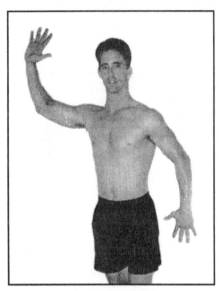

Figure 1

Right hand at 90° angle, facing upward
Left hand at 90° angle, facing downward.

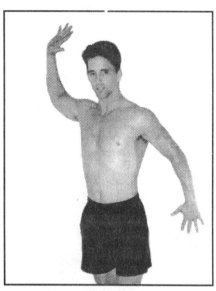

Figure 2

- Stretch both hands backward at the same time until your chest is tight;
- Release; Return to original position.

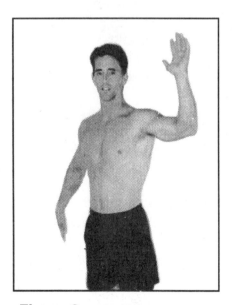

Figure 3

[Reverse of Figure 1]
Left hand at 90° angle, facing upward
Right hand at 90° angle, facing downward.

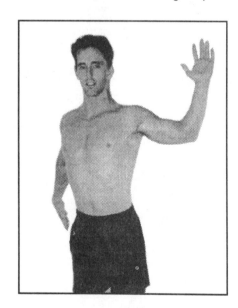

Figure 4

- Stretch both hands backward at the same time until your chest is tight;
- Release; Return to original position.

A. Upper Body Stretches

8. Press, Press — Fling

This is a good stretch for the chest that can be used before and after the push-up segment.

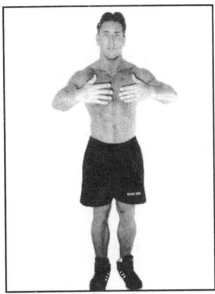

Figure 1

Bring hands in front of your chest, with palms facing inward.

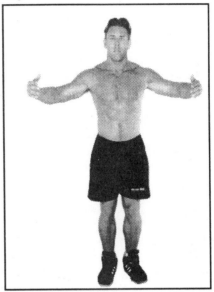

Figure 2

- In one fluid motion, extend hands and arms outward, no further than shown above.
- Maintain hands and arms in a half circle configuration through the movement.

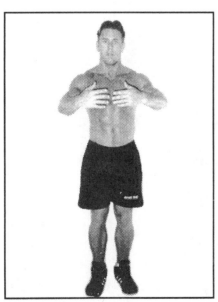

Figure 3

Bring hands and arms back to the original position shown in Figure 1.

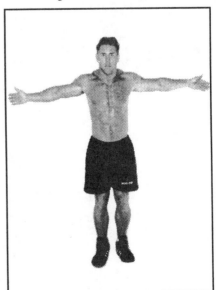

Figure 4

Extend arms out and back as far as possible, but release hands at the very end of the motion, so that your arms are completely straight.

B. Lower Body Stretches

9. Thigh Stretch - Standing

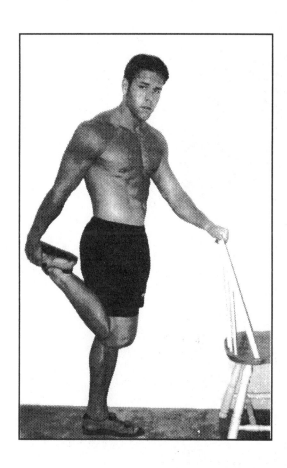

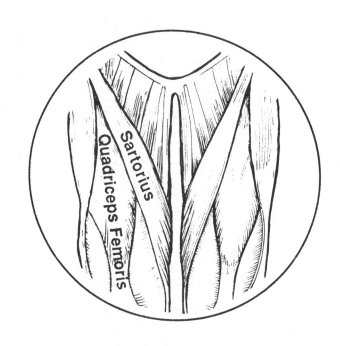

Sartorius

Quadriceps Femoris

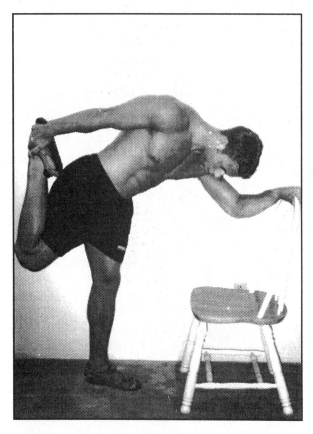

Figure 1 *(Above)*

- Place one hand on anything stable enough to support you.
- Take your other hand and grab your toes on the same side.

Figure 2 *(Rght)*

- Pull your toes up behind you, stretching your thigh.
- Switch sides.

B. Lower Body Stretches

10. Calf Stretch

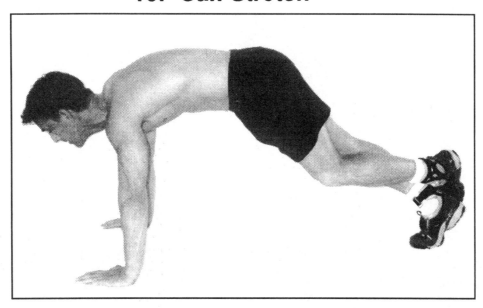

Figure 1

- Assume the push-up position.
- Place your left foot over your right heel, as shown in Figure 2.
- In a slow movement, try placing your right heel flat on the ground.
- If the tightness in your calf becomes painful, stop and ease up on the pressure.
- Switch to the other leg.

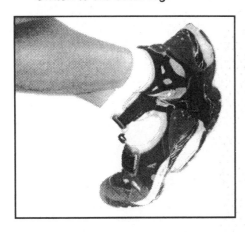

Figure 2

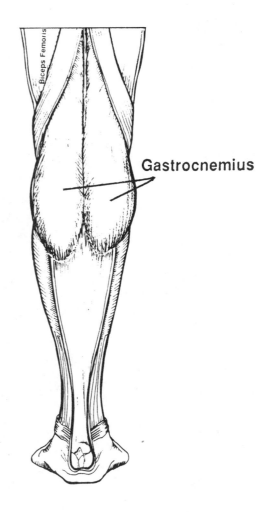

B. Lower Body Stretches

11. Sit Down Bend-Over

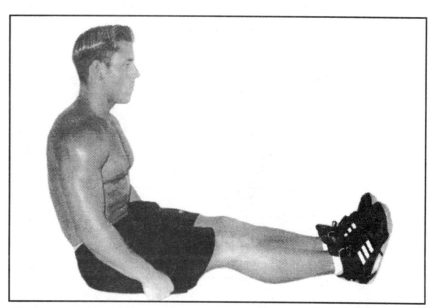

Figure 1

- Sit on the ground. Keep your legs together.
- The key factor is to keep your legs straight, with a slight bend in your knees.
- Maintain a straight back throughout the stretch.

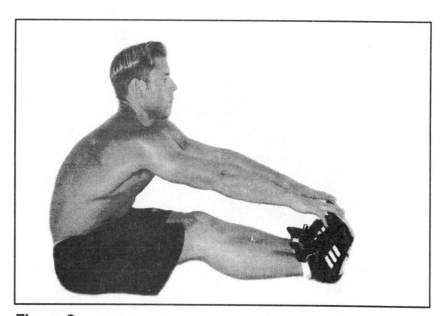

Figure 2

- Lean over and try to touch your toes with your hands. (O.K. to touch toes, but do not grab and pull back.)
- Hold for 10-15 seconds; Release.

B. Lower Body Stretches

12. Hurdler's Stretch

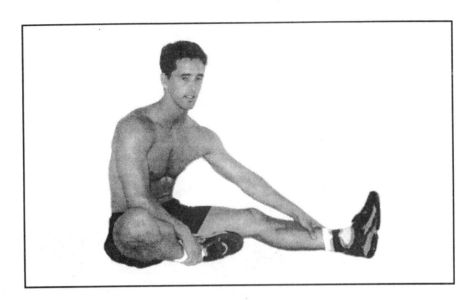

Figure 1

- Sit down.
- Bend your right leg inward, so that your right foot is flat against the inside of your left knee or thigh.

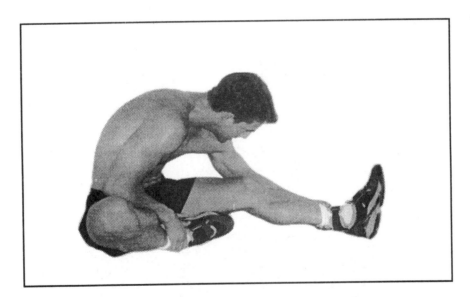

Figure 2

- Place your right hand on your right foot [or right ankle; assume the most comfortable position].
- Lean over toward your left foot. Try to touch your chest to your left knee.
- Switch legs.

B. Lower Body Stretches

13. ITB Stretch

This stretch is great for loosening a tight lower back and for stretching the ITB (iliotibial) tendon, which runs from your hip to your knee.

Figure 1

- Sit down.
- Keep your left leg straight.
- Place your right foot next to your left knee.

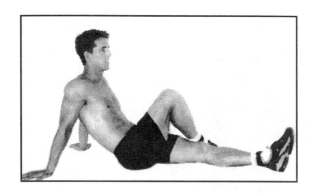

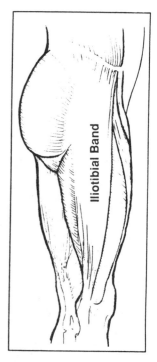

Iliotibial Band

Figure 2

- Wrap your right knee with left arm, followed by placing your right hand on your left elbow.
- Slowly bring your right knee toward your chest, holding it for 15 to 30 seconds.

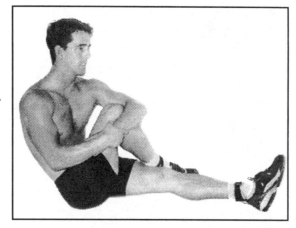

Figure 3

- Next, place the outer part of your left elbow against the outer part of your right knee, while reaching back with your right hand.
- Place your right hand on the ground, about a foot behind your lower back.
- Slowly twist to the right while pushing your right knee to the left.
- Hold this position 15 seconds.
- Switch to the other leg.

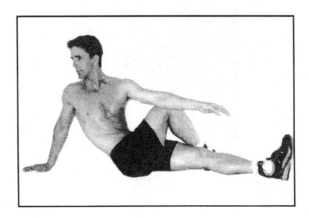

B. Lower Body Stretches

14. Butterfly Stretch

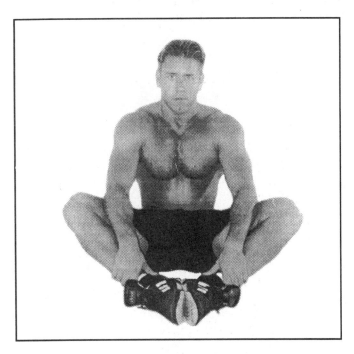

Figure 1

- Sit down.

- Make a diamond shape with your legs.

- Place your heels together.

- Grab your ankles and slowly bring your heels toward you until they are close to six inches from you.

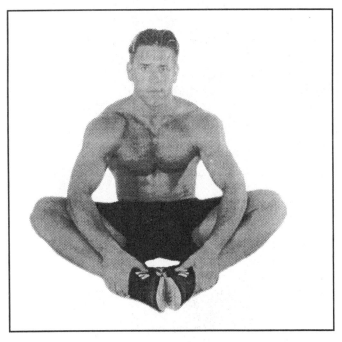

Figure 2

- Put pressure on your knees by placing your elbows on your knees, pushing them downward.

- Hold this position for 15 seconds.

- Release and relax for 10 seconds.

- Repeat this process again, 3 or 4 times.

B. Lower Body Stretches

15. Trunk Extensions

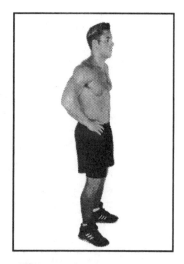

Figure 1

- Stand up straight, with your feet shoulder-width apart.
- Place your hands on your waist.
- Keep your legs straight.

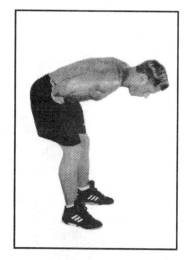

Figure 2

- Lean forward as far as you can; Hold for 15 seconds.
- Straighten back up.

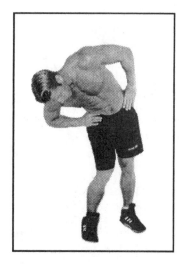

Figure 3

- Now lean to your right side;
- Hold for 15 seconds.

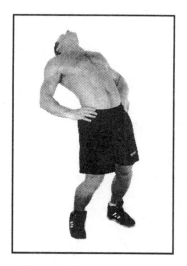

Figure 4

Lean to your back; Thrust your hips forward and keep your hands on your waist;
- Hold for 15 seconds.

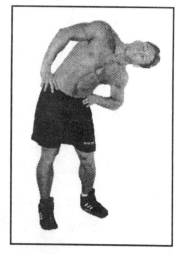

Figure 5

- Now lean to your left side;
- Hold for 15 seconds.

Maintain knees bent to prevent hyperextending your back.
The first repetition should be slow. Following repetitions can be more fluid.
You will soon be able to rotate smoothly through each phase of this exercise.

B. Lower Body Stretches

16. Cobra Stretch

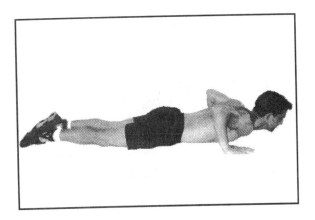

Figure 1

- Lay flat on your stomach; legs together and straight.
- Place your hands [flat, palms down] next to your chest; Look straight ahead.

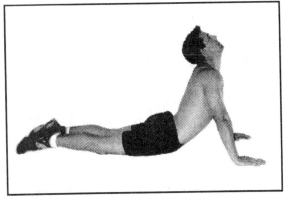

Figure 2

Raise your upper torso and rotate your head back.

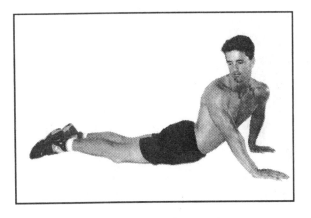

Figure 3

Lean toward the right, dipping your left shoulder.

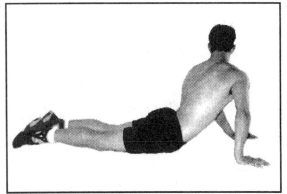

Figure 4

Now lean toward the left, dipping your right shoulder.

B. Lower Body Stretches

17. Hamstring Stretch

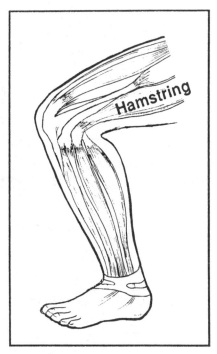

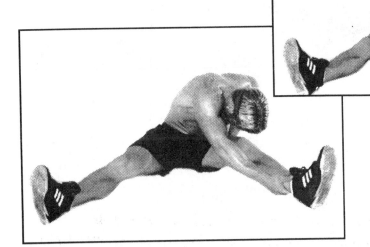

Figure 1 *(Above)*

Assume spread-eagle position.

Figure 2 *(left)*

- Reach over with your right hand and grab your left ankle.
- Bring your chest down to your knee.

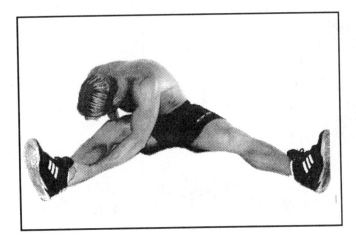

Figure 3

[Reverse of Figure 2]

- Reach over with your left hand and grab your right ankle.
- Bring your chest down to your knee.

B. Lower Body Stretches

18. Inner Thigh Stretch

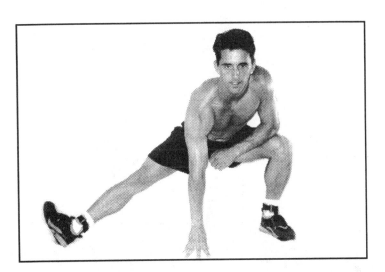

Figure 1

- Place your right hand on the ground for support.

- Extend your right foot and leg outward; keep your toes pointed up.

- Lean toward your left knee, while placing your left elbow on your thigh for support. [Do not allow your left knee to go past a 90° angle.]

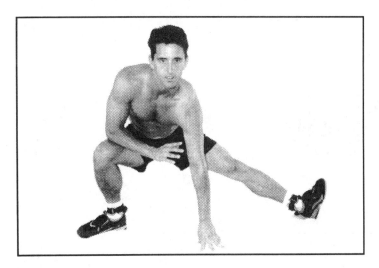

Figure 2

- Place your left hand on the ground for support.

- Extend your left foot and leg outward; keep your toes pointed up.

- Lean toward your right knee, while placing your right elbow on your thigh for support. [Do not allow your left knee to go past a 90° angle.]

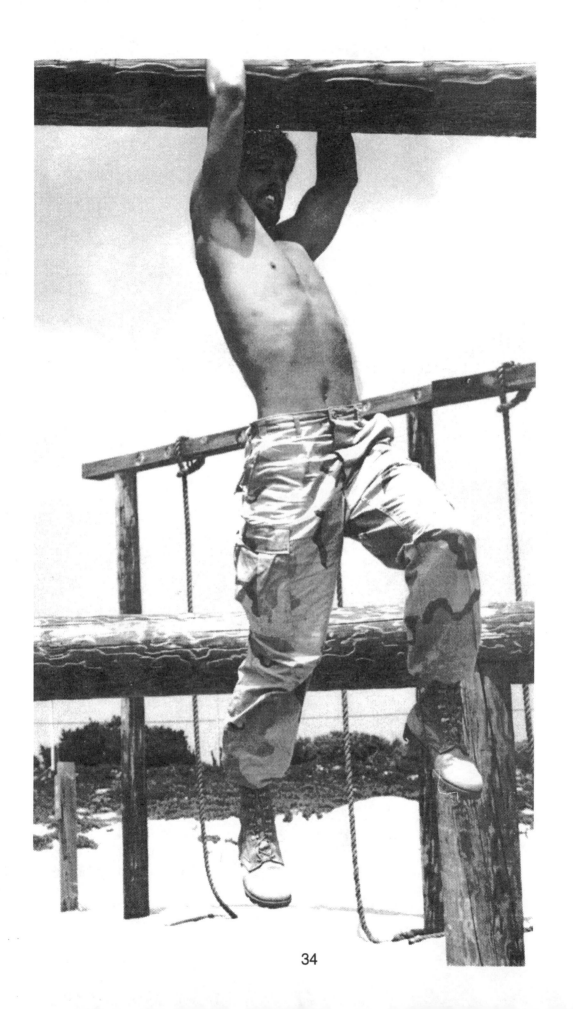

II. Upper Body Workout

II.   Upper Body Workout

he upper body is an area where, besides your abdominals, you will see the quickest results. Just as you stretch during the stomach and leg exercises, it is extremely important to stretch *throughout* your upper body routine. Using the upper body stretches I've shown you will allow you to pump out more repetitions.

I have divided the Upper Body Workout into three sections because of the rate of growth and change these muscles go through. **Do the exercises in the order I have written for maximum benefit.** The pull-ups [page 38] and bar dips [page 45] are first, followed by push-ups [page 46] . This order will "burn out" your upper body before the push-ups, which will lead to a more effective push-up session. The Upper Body Workout utilizes the pyramid system (ascending repetitions, followed by corresponding descending repetitions). As an example, let's go through the Upper Body Workout - Beginner Program, week one [page 50] .

1. First, do 1 regular pull-up.
    Drop off the pull-up bar.
    Rest 15 seconds.

2. Next, do 2 regular pull-ups.
    Drop off the pull-up bar.
    Rest 15 seconds.
    Then do 1 more pull-up, drop off the bar,
    and rest 15 seconds.

3. Now do the reverse grip pull-ups [page 41],
    utilizing the same format for these [and following
    pull-ups].

After you are done with the pull-ups, move to the bar dips.

- Do 4 sets of 5 dips, with a 15 - 30 second rest
  in-between sets.

Finally, move to the push-ups.

- Do 2 regular push-ups.
  Rest 15 seconds.

- Do 4 regular push-ups.
  Rest 15 seconds.

- Do 2 regular push-ups.
  Rest 15 seconds.

Now move to the tricep push-ups [page 47], utilizing the same format for these and the rest of the pull-ups.

Do not — *I repeat* — do not sacrifice form for repetition.

Just because you are one repetition away from finally reaching the advanced level does not mean you may break form and raise your buttocks into the air, or fail to touch your chest on the ground. Do not cheat yourself. You have plenty of time.

When To Advance

You do not have to reach the next level in all exercises before advancing. If you can perform intermediate level push-ups, but only beginner level pull-ups, that's fine.

And don't forget—your greatest gain in fitness and strength will occur when you use proper form.

Always do as much as you can without injuring yourself. The average person will advance faster in push-ups and bar dips than in pull-ups. It all depends on each person's individual strength and fitness level.

Continually strive to increase your repetitions. After the first week, increase your push-ups. Then, after three weeks, move up in pull-ups. By the fifth week you should be doing four sets of eight dips. Once you reach your fifth week, you will be able to increase your repetitions weekly. This will become quite challenging. And don't forget—your greatest gain in fitness and strength will occur when you use proper form.

It's time to go to work.

Good luck!

II. Upper Body Workout

19. Regular Pull-Up

Works back and side muscle groups

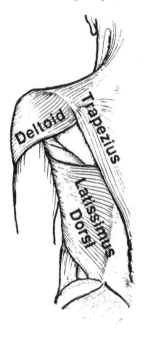

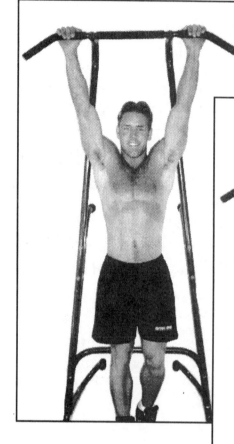

Figure 1

This exercise can only be performed on a strong pull-up bar. Grasp the pull-up bar so that your hands are shoulder-width apart.

Figure 2

• Raise your body up so that your chin is at or above the pull-up bar.

• Lower your body *slowly*, to prevent injury.

• When you are fully extended down, start back up again.

Training Tip

19.   Pull-Up (by yourself)

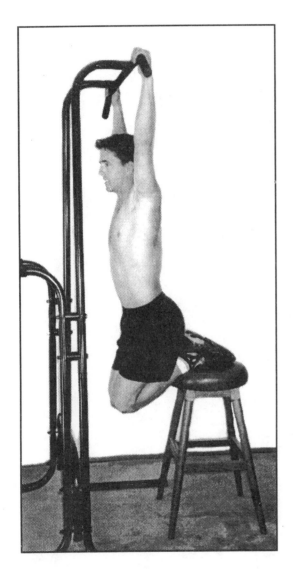

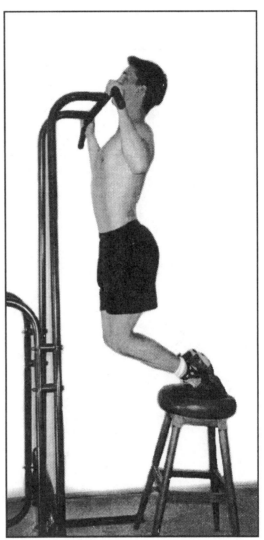

Figure 1

Take an ordinary stool and place it below you, so that you can rest your feet on top. Do not use stool to support you, it is just a helping tool.

Figure 2

- Use only your thigh muscles to elevate your upper body.

- Just remember to release your feet before dropping off the pull-up bar, or landing will be a very unpleasant experience...

Training Tip

19. Pull-Up (with a partner)

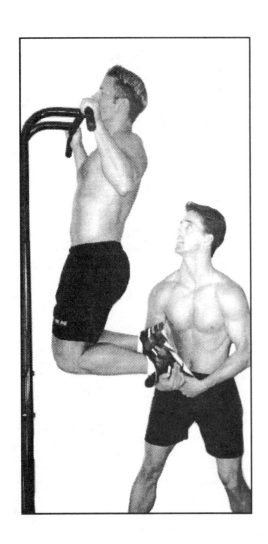 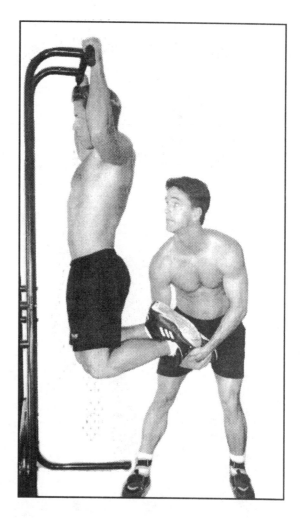

Figure 1
Starting Position

This photograph demonstrates
the proper pull-up technique.

Figure 2
Ending Position

The key to this technique is to have
your partner hold your feet steady at
a 90° angle while you use your thigh
muscles to elevate your body.

20. Reverse Grip Pull-Up

This exercise will work your biceps and upper back.

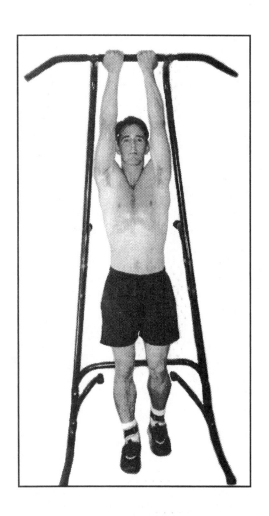
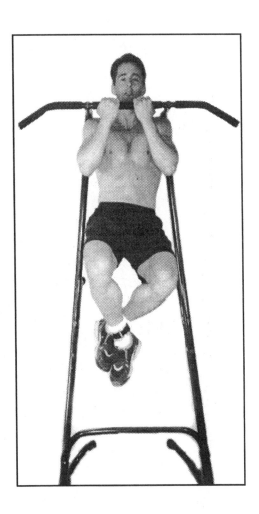

Figure 1

Place your hands on the pull-up bar as shown [2" to 3 " apart], palms facing you.

Figure 2

- Pull yourself up until your chin is above the bar.

- Lower yourself down slowly, then start back up again.

21. Close Grip Pull-Ups

This exercise will work your forearms, triceps, and upper back.

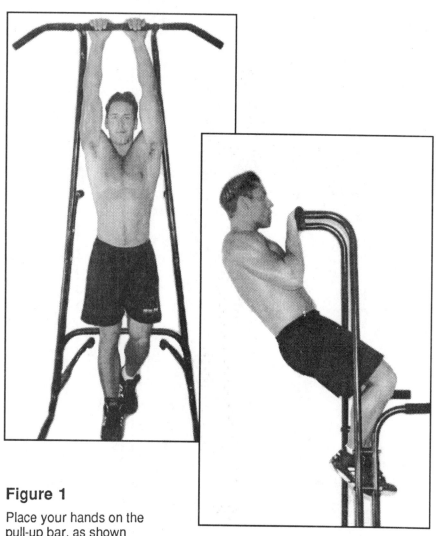

Figure 1

Place your hands on the
pull-up bar, as shown
[2" to 3" apart], with your
palms facing away from you.

Figure 2

- Pull yourself up so that
  your chin is above bar.

- Lower your body *slowly,*
  to prevent injury.

- When you are fully extended
  down, start back up again.

II. Upper Body Workout

22. Behind the Neck Pull-Up

This is an incredible exercise for the upper back and lats. If you've ever noticed, every Navy SEAL has incredible back development. This exercise is a major reason why. This is also one of the most difficult exercises to perform.

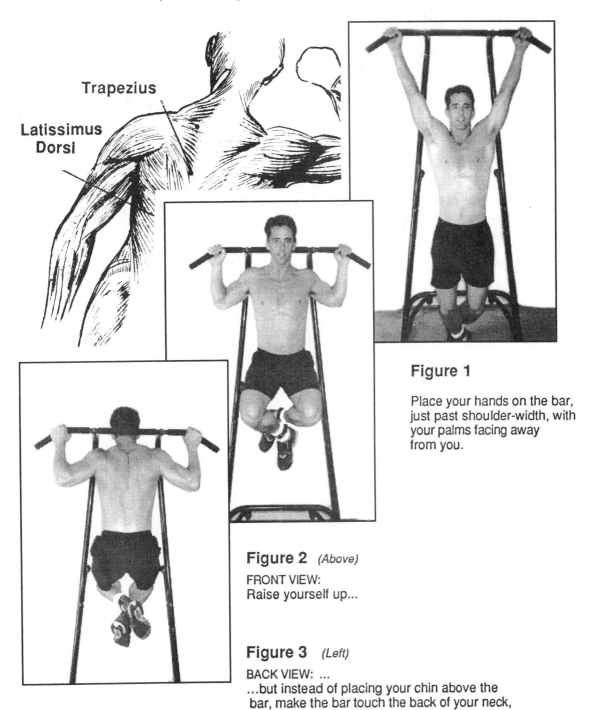

Trapezius

Latissimus
Dorsi

Figure 1

Place your hands on the bar, just past shoulder-width, with your palms facing away from you.

Figure 2 *(Above)*
FRONT VIEW:
Raise yourself up...

Figure 3 *(Left)*
BACK VIEW: ...
...but instead of placing your chin above the bar, make the bar touch the back of your neck, as close to your shoulders as possible.

II. Upper Body Workout

23. Commando Pull-Up

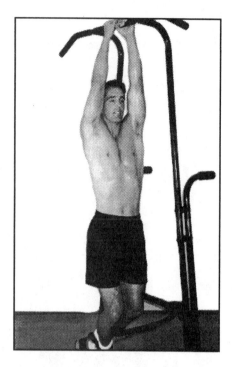

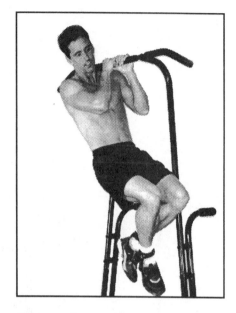

Figure 1

Facing sideways, grab the bar, placing the thumb of your left hand directly next to the pinkie of your right hand...

Figure 2

Pull yourself up, touching your right shoulder to the bar.

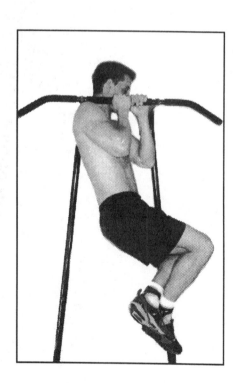

Figure 3 *(Right)*

- Lower yourself down slowly, then pull yourself back up again, so the bar touches your left shoulder. That counts as one repetition.

- Do not jerk yourself up during this or any pull-up exercise since that will not isolate any muscle group. Jerking yourself up relies too much on your body's momentum, rather than muscle performance.

II. Upper Body Workout

24.　Bar Dip

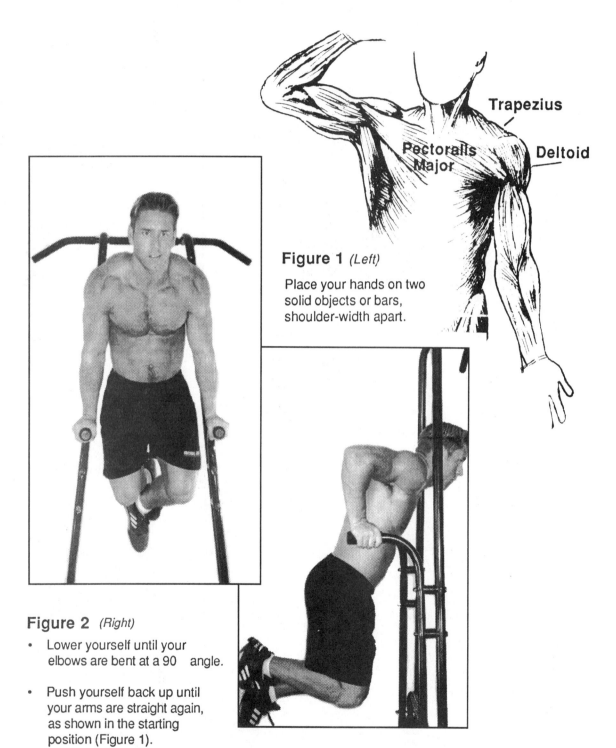

Figure 1 *(Left)*

Place your hands on two solid objects or bars, shoulder-width apart.

Trapezius

Pectoralis Major

Deltoid

Figure 2 *(Right)*

- Lower yourself until your elbows are bent at a 90 angle.

- Push yourself back up until your arms are straight again, as shown in the starting position (Figure 1).

II. Upper Body Workout

25. Push-Up

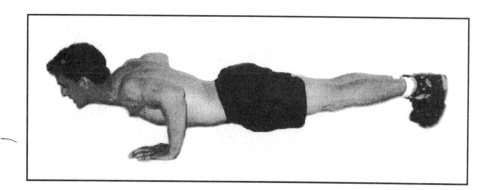

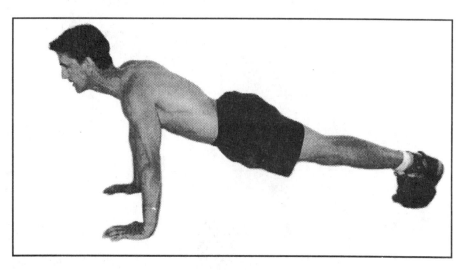

Deltoid

Pectoralis Major

Bicep

Tricep

Figure 1

- Assume the standard push-up position.
- Keep your arms slightly outside of shoulder-width.
- Keep your body perfectly parallel to the ground.

Figure 2

- Bend your elbows and lower yourself until your chest *(lightly)* touches the ground.
- Immediately push yourself back up to the starting position.
- Fully extend your arms when coming back up. ***No cheating!***

Do not rest your chest on the ground !

During SEAL training that was a BIG mistake! If you tried to rest your chest on the ground, or if you were not going all the way down, the instructor would make you stop and start all over again—which often resulted in having to do triple the original amount!

II. Upper Body Workout

26. Tricep Push-Up

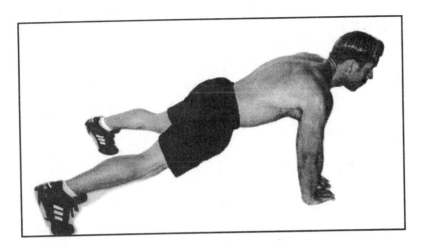

Figure 1

Similar to a regular push-up, except spread your feet shoulder-width apart.

Figure 2   *[right]*

Place your hands together, making a diamond shape with your thumbs and index fingers.

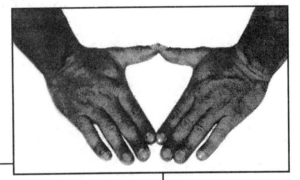

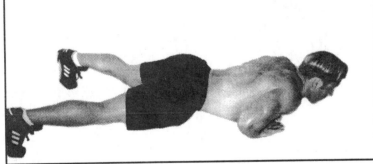

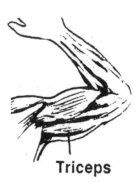

Triceps

Figure 3

- Lower yourself so that the diamond shape of your hands touches your lower chest, as shown above.
- Raise your body back up to the starting position.
- **Reminder: Do not rest your chest on the ground!**

II. Upper Body Workout

27. Dive Bomber

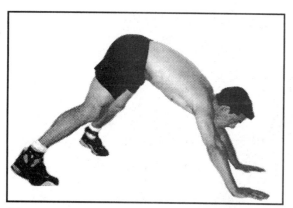

Figure 1

- Assume the push-up position. Spread your feet shoulder-width apart, with your buttocks high in the air.

- Bring your feet 12" - 18" toward your hands.

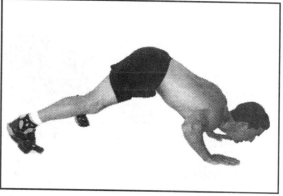

Figure 2

- Push your head toward the ground.

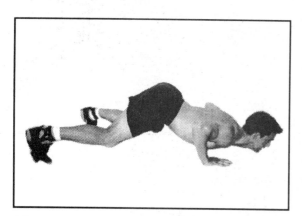

Figure 3

- Now pretend you are trying to put your head through a hole at the bottom of a fence...

- Maintain that position for 2-3 seconds.

- In the same fluid motion, bring your body back to the original position.

II. Upper Body Workout

28. Wide Angle Push-Up

This allows you to work your chest muscles at a different angle. Working your muscles from different angles will increase muscle strength and development.

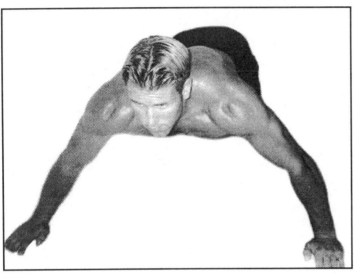

Figure 1

Same as Exercise #19, Regular Push-Up, except extend your arms farther out, as shown above.

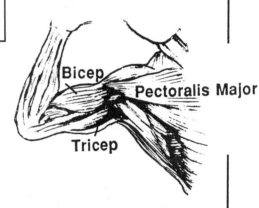

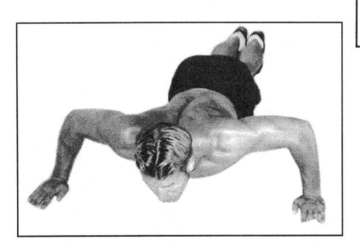

Figure 2

Perform the push-up in this position.

II. Upper Body Workout

Beginner

Instructions:

l.   Find the columns below headed **"Exercise"** and "**Repetitions.**"

2.   Under "Exercise" find **"A. Pull-Ups"** and go down to **"1. Regular."**

3.   Under "Repetitions" see **"Week 1"**.

4.   The repetitions required for this exercise in Week 1 are: **"1 - 2 - 1"**.

5.   The repetitions are completed as follows:

> Perform **1** regular pull-up, drop off the bar; rest 15 seconds;
> Perform **2** regular pull-ups, drop off the bar; rest 15 seconds;
> Perform **1** regular pull-up; drop off the bar.

6.   **It is important that you perform all repetitions and 15-second rests for all all exercises in this book. Perform exercises exactly in the order specified.**

7.   Exercise repetitions in this format (example: 1-Warm-up, **2-Peak**, and 1-Cool Down) are significantly more beneficial to your muscular strength and development than performing other random exercise patterns.

Exercise   Repetitions

A. Pull-Ups

		Week 1	Weeks 3 - 5
1.	Regular	1 - 2 - 1	1 - 2 - 3 - 2 - 1
2.	Reverse	1 - 2 - 1	1 - 2 - 3 - 2 - 1
3.	Close Grip	1 - 2 - 1	1 - 2 - 3 - 2 - 1
4.	Behind the Neck	1 - 2 - 1	1 - 2 - 3 - 2 - 1
5.	Regular Pull-Up	1 - 2 - 1	1 - 2 - 3 - 2 - 1

B. Bar Dips   4 Sets of 5

C. Push-Ups

		Week 1	Weeks 2 - 4	Week 5
1.	Regular	2 - 4 - 2	2 - 4 - 4 -2	4 - 6 - 4 - 2 - 2
2.	Tricep	2 - 4 - 2	2 - 4 - 4 -2	4 - 6 - 4 - 2 - 2
3.	Dive Bomber	2 - 4 - 2	2 - 4 - 4 -2	4 - 6 - 4 - 2 - 2
4.	Wide Angle	2 - 4 - 2	2 - 4 - 4 -2	4 - 6 - 4 - 2 - 2

•   Perform the Upper Body Workout - Beginner program (A, B & C, above) every Monday, Wednesday and Friday

II. Upper Body Workout
Intermediate

Complete the Intermediate Workout five times a week, as follows:

To Start: Perform this program (A, B & C) every Monday, Wednesday and Friday – for 4 weeks.

Progress: After 4 weeks, advance to 5 times a week.

Perform stretches before and after each workout section:

Upper Body Stretches: Section I - Part A, pages 16 through 23.
Single Arm Stretch: page 17.

Exercise   Repetitions

A.   Pull-Ups

  1.   Regular   1 - 2 - 3 - 4 - **5** - 4 - 3 - 2 - 1

  2.   Reverse   1 - 2 - 3 - **4** - 3 - 2 - 1

  3.   Close Grip   1 - 2 - 3 - **4** - 3 - 2 - 1

  4.   Behind-the-Neck   1 - 2 - 3 - **4** - 3 - 2 - 1

  5.   Commando   1 - **2** - **2** - 1

B.   Bar Dip   4 Sets of 15

C.   Push-Ups

  1.   Regular   2 - 4 - 6 - 8 - **10** - 8 - 6 - 4 - 2

  2.   Tricep   2 - 4 - 6 - **8** - 6 - 4 - 2

  3.   Dive Bomber   2 - 4 - 6 - **8** - 6 - 4 - 2

  4.   Wide Angle   2 - 4 - 6 - **8** - 6 - 4 - 2

II. Upper Body Workout
Advanced

Complete the Advanced Workout five times a week, as follows:

To Start: Perform this program (A, B & C) every Monday, Wednesday and Friday — for 4 weeks.

Progress: After 4 weeks, advance to 5 times a week.

Perform stretches before and after each workout section.

Upper Body Stretches: Section I - Part A, pages 16 through 23.
Single Arm Stretch: page 17.

Exercise   ## Repetitions

A. Pull-Ups

1.	Regular	1 - 2 - 3 - 4 - 5 - 6 - 7 - **8** - 7 - 6 - 5 - 4 - 3 - 2 - 1
2.	Reverse	1 - 2 - 3 - 4 - 5 - **6** - 5 - 4 - 3 - 2 - 1
3.	Close Grip	1 - 2 - 3 - 4 - 5 - **6** - 5 - 4 - 3 - 2 - 1
4.	Behind the Neck	1 - 2 - 3 - 4 - 5 - **6** - 5 - 4 - 3 - 2 - 1
5.	Commando	1 - 2 - 3 - **4** - 3 - 2 - 1

B. Bar Dips   4 Sets of 20

C. Push-Ups

1.	Regular	2 - 4 - 6 - 8 - 10 - 12 - **14** - 12 - 10 - 8 - 6 - 4 - 2
2.	Tricep	2 - 4 - 6 - 8 - 10 - **12** - 10 - 8 - 6 - 4 - 2
3.	Dive Bomber	2 - 4 - 6 - 8 - 10 - **12** - 10 - 8 - 6 - 4 - 2
4.	Wide Angle	2 - 4 - 6 - 8 - 10 - **12** - 10 - 8 - 6 - 4

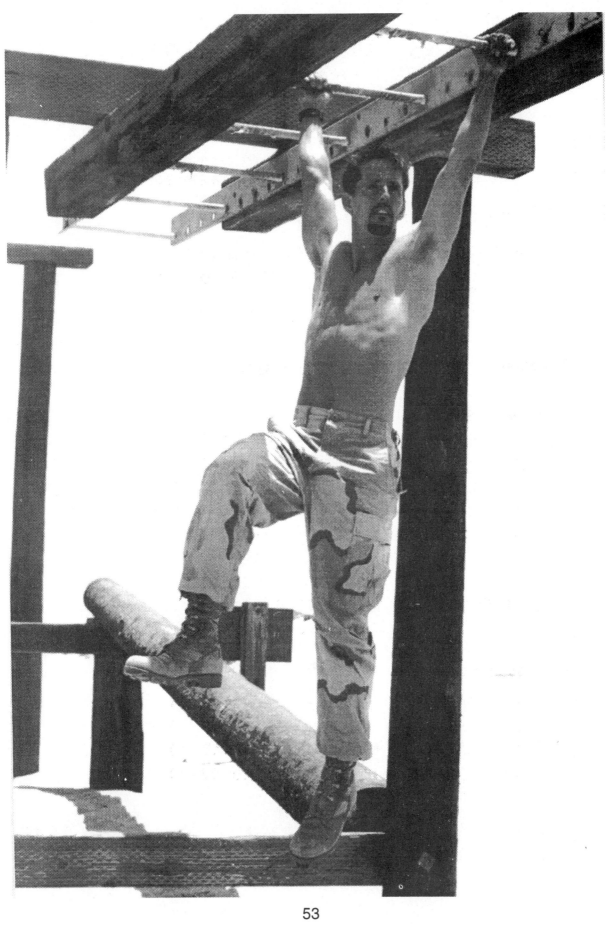

III. Lower Body Workout

III. Lower Body Workout

During SEAL training I had to do thousands and thousands of sit-ups. Without proper form, I would not have been able to keep up or maintain a healthy back.

Pay strict attention to these instructions and use the pictures to help you learn proper form. Doing these exercises *as instructed* will get your abs into phenomenal condition, and will also keep you from injuring yourself.

In-between Lower Body Workout exercises, it is wise to use the Cobra Stretch to loosen up your abdominals. Perform this stretch every third exercise. [Cobra Stretch, see page 31].

Never be satisfied with the fitness level you are working on — until you reach your final goal. Continually push yourself past your limits.

At the end of each week increase your repetitions in increments of five. If one week is not enough time to reach your goals, then increase every two weeks. Keep increasing until you reach sixty. When you are comfortable with 60 and ready to go on to 65 — *stop!*

Now you are ready to move on to the advanced stage.

This is the same as the beginning of the intermediate stage, except you perform two sets of 35 repetitions each—instead of one set of 60. Once again, continue to increase by increments of five until you reach 60 again. At this point, increase your sets to three.

Never be satisfied with the fitness level you are working on, until you reach your final goal. Continually push yourself past your limits. Only when you push yourself will you be capable of achieving the results and fitness level you desire.

Let's get started

III.   Lower Body Workout

29. Sit-Up

While doing sit-ups, remember these points to avoid injuries:

1. Do not place your hands behind your neck because this causes too much strain on your back and legs.

2. Avoid bringing your chest up to your thighs. This also puts too much strain on your back.

3. Do not rock during your sit-ups.

4. Perform each sit-up with strict movements to isolate your abdominals.

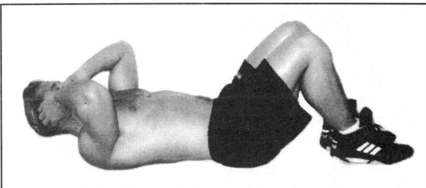

Figure 1

- Place your hands so they are barely touching your ears.

- Bend your knees and place your feet 12-18 inches from your buttocks. Maintain this distance throughout the exercise.

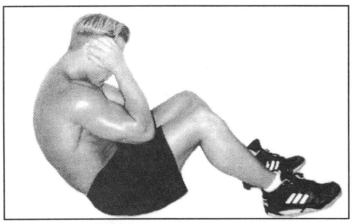

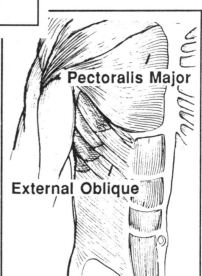

Figure 2

- Bring yourself up so your elbows touch your thighs.

- Keep your abdominal muscles tight; use the full force of your stomach muscle to raise your upper body.

Training Tip

Proper Hand Position for
29.   Sit-Up

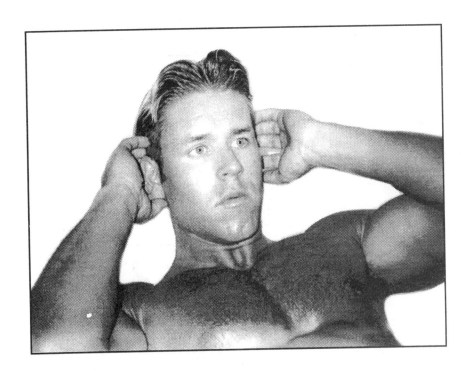

Figure 1

- Fingers should be gently touching the outer part of the ears.
- Do NOT place your hands behind your neck, as this will cause injury to the neck.

III. Lower Body Workout

30. Half Sit-Up

While doing sit-ups, remember this important point:
Be sure to lower your upper body *slowly* to avoid injuring your back.

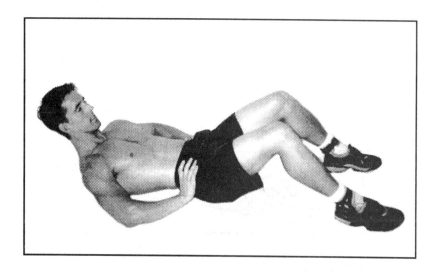

Figure 1
- Assume the position shown above.
- Bend your knees as shown; place your feet 2 to 3 feet from your buttocks.

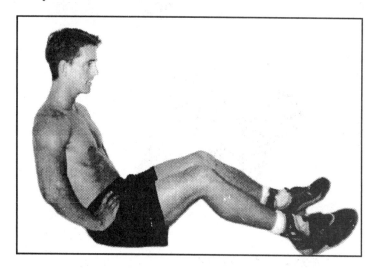

Figure 2
- Place your hands on your waist and bring your upper body up halfway, or 45°.
- Do not go up any further than a 45° angle.
- Lower yourself down and raise yourself back up to a 45° angle.
- This is one repetition.

III. Lower Body Workout

31. Hand-to-Toe

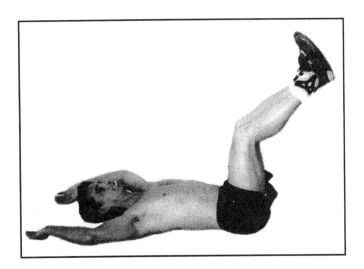

Figure 1

Lay on the ground on your back, with your arms over your head, and raise your legs at a 90° angle.

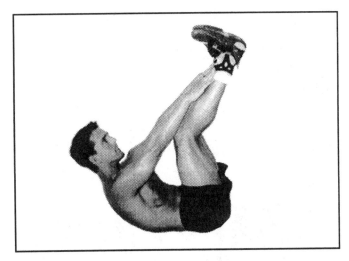

Figure 2

- Raise up your upper body and try to touch your toes.

- Keep your legs as straight as possible throughout the entire motion; your legs will bend slightly, naturally.

- It is extremely important to raise your shoulder blades off the ground, or you will defeat the purpose of this exercise.

- It is OK if you can not touch your toes. Just go for your knees. As your physical fitness and flexibility improves, go for your toes.

32. Crunch

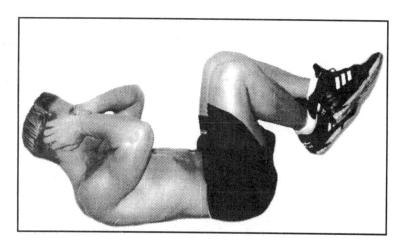

Figure 1

- Lay on your back and raise your knees to a 90° angle.

- Maintain this position while placing your hands in the sit-up position. Once again, your hands should barely touch your ears to avoid added stress to the neck.

- Do not allow your shoulder to touch the ground.

- Isolate your stomach muscles (tight) during the entire movement.

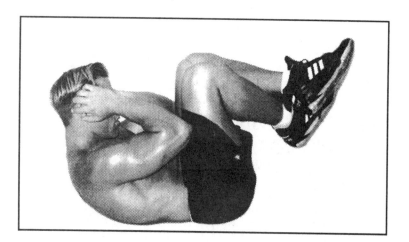

Figure 2

- Raise your upper body toward your thighs, so your elbows touch them; using your abdominal muscles topull you up.

- Once you have reached your thighs, lower yourself down with control.

60

33. Side Sit-Up

This is an excellent exercise for the right side abdominal muscles.

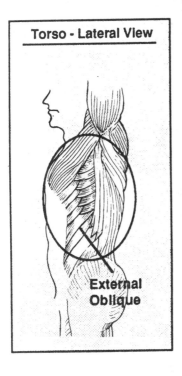

Torso - Lateral View

External Oblique

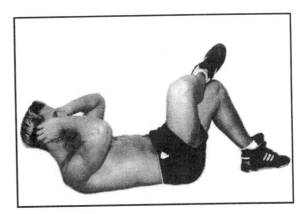

Figure 1

- Lay down in the sit-up position and place your right ankle on your left knee, so that your right knee is perpendicular to your body.

- Place your hands in the standard position, applying little or no pressure on your ears.

- Do not allow your shoulder to touch the ground.

- Maintain your stomach muscles tight during this entire movement.

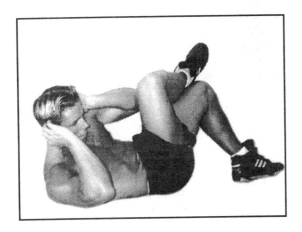

Figure 2

Raise your upper body so that your left elbow touches your right knee, and then slowly bring yourself back down.

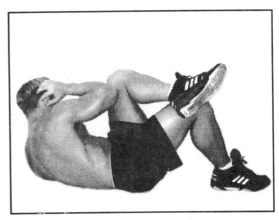

Figure 3

Once you have finished with the left side, switch legs and work your right side.

34. Oblique

Technique is really important is this exercise, in order to get the full effect.

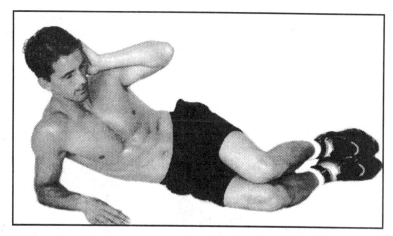

Figure 1

- Lay on your side, keeping your knees and feet together.
- Your upper body should be propped up on your eblow.
- Place your opposite hand by your ear, in the same manner as instructed for sit-ups.

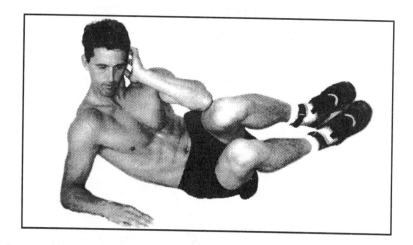

Figure 2

- Here is the key part! Raise your feet straight up, as if someone has tied a string to your feet and is pulling it up and down.
- Curl your upper body until your elbow is touching your knees. Slowly lower your upper body down.
- Once you have completed the recommended repetitions, switch sides and begin the process over again.
- Raise your knees.   Do not curl or bend your knees toward your chest.

III. Lower Body Workout

35. Flutter Kick

- Do not be concerned about speed. This is a technique exercise.

- This exercise is to be done in a "four count" mode. As each foot is raised up to the 36 inch mark, start counting "one, two. . ." On the fourth mark, count the cumulative total.

    For example: *1-2-3-* **1**, *1-2-3-* **2**, *1-2-3-* **3**, *1-2-3-* **4**.

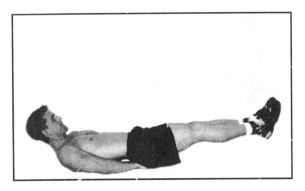

Figure 1

- Lay on your back and place your hands under your buttocks, palms down. This position will give your hips support.

- Raise both feet off the ground 6 inches, keeping your legs straight.

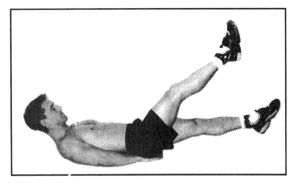

Figure 2

- Raise your right foot, then lower it back down to the starting position.

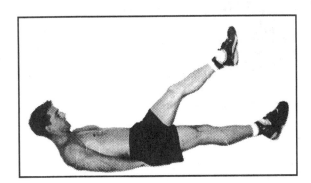

Figure 3

As you do so, raise your left foot 36 inches off the ground.

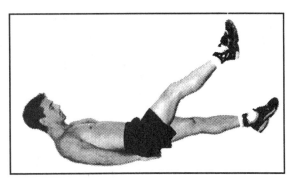

Figure 4

- Bring your left foot back down and raise your right foot back up to the 36" mark.

- Continue alternating in a fluid motion.

In the advanced section, when doing higher reps, it is recommended that you do this exercise 3 times a week or every-other day.

III. Lower Body Workout

36. Leg Raise

Remember to isolate your abdominal muscles when performing this exercise.

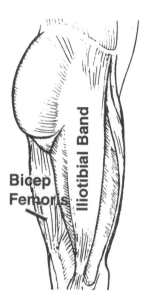

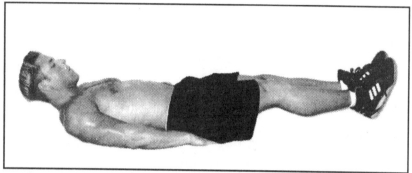

Figure 1

- Lay down on your back, placing your hands under your buttocks, palms down. This will give your back support.
- Raise your feet 6" off the ground, heels together.

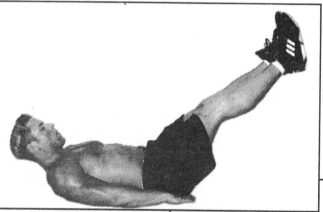

Figure 2

Raise your legs up 36" heels together, as shown.

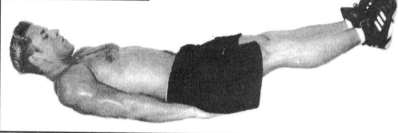

Figure 3

- Lower your legs until both feet are again 6" off the ground.
- This is one repetition.

If you are new at exercising, or it has been awhile, then it is recommended that this exercise be done with one leg on the ground to relieve tension on the lower back. Once one repetition is finished, then switch legs.

III. Lower Body Workout

37. Cutting Edge

This is an excellent lower abdominal exercise.

Figure 1

- Lay down on your back, placing your hands under your buttocks, palms down. This will give your back support.

- Raise your legs up, heels together, about 6 " off the ground.

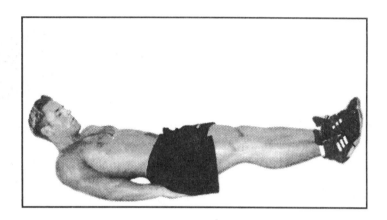

Figure 2

- Spread your legs apart to 48 ", or just past shoulder-width, and bring them back together. This is one repetition.

- Continue in this manner until you have completed the required repetitions.

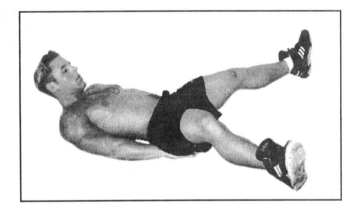

Figure 3

Then bring your feet together again one last time, and lower both feet to the ground.

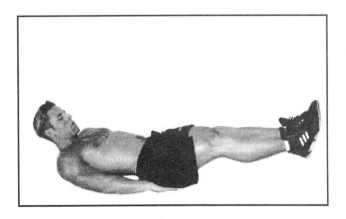

III. Lower Body Workout

38. Knee Bend

There is a point in this exercise which allows you to keep your balance easier. Extend your legs out straight, heels on the ground. Begin leaning back with your hands by your ears. The moment your feet begin to rise off the ground, you've found your "equilibrium point." This is the best position in which to perform this exercise.

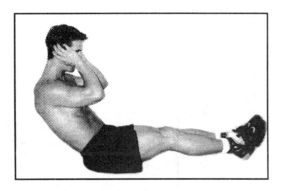

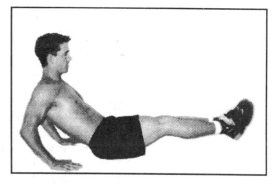

Figure 1

- Sit on the ground with your torso at a 45° angle.

- Raise your feet up 6 inches.

- Place your hands by your ears, as if in the sit-up position.

Figure 2

If it is too difficult for you to keep your balance, put your hands on the ground for support.

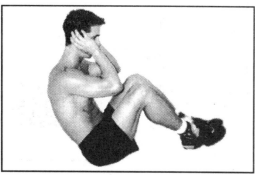

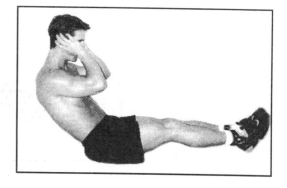

Figure 3

- Bring your knees toward your chest smooth, fluid motion.

- **Do not allow your feet to touch the ground!**

Figure 4

Extend your legs back out in a again until they are straight.

[See figure 1]

III. Lower Body Workout

39. Helen Keller

This exercise requires a lot of balance and control with your abdominal muscles. Only with time and practice will this exercise become more efficient and smooth.

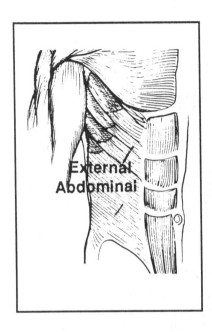

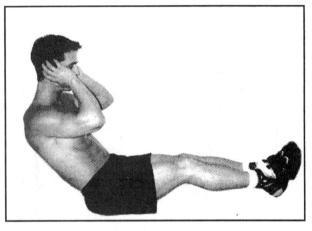

Figure 1

- Sit on the ground with your back at a 45° angle.
- Raise your legs 3 inches off the ground.

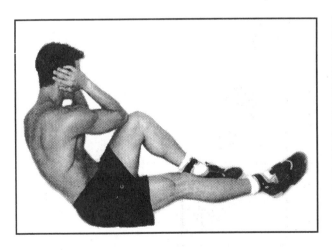

Figure 2

- Raise your left knee toward you, making a 90° angle from your hip.
- Now bring your right elbow across your body and touch your left kneecap.
- Then lower your left knee and...

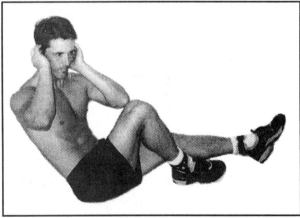

Figure 3

... raise your right knee, touching your right knee with your left elbow.

- Continue exercising in this manner, alternating knees.

40. Hanging Knee-Up

You must have access to a pull-up bar to perform this exercise.

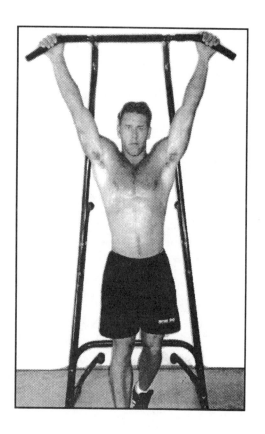

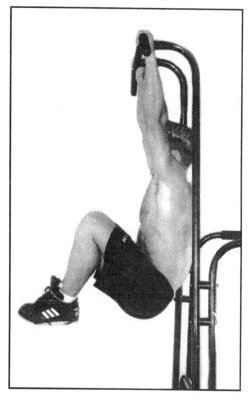

Figure 1

- Assume the starting position shown above.

- The object is to keep your upper body stable while performing this exercise.

Figure 2

- Raise your knees up to your chest, so that your thighs are flush against your stomach.

- Slowly lower your knees until your legs are straight down.

- **To avoid putting too much strain on your back, do not drop your legs down quickly.**

41. Hanging Leg-Up

To do this exercise you must have access to a pull-up bar. I know this is a difficult exercise, so just take your time and do the best you can!

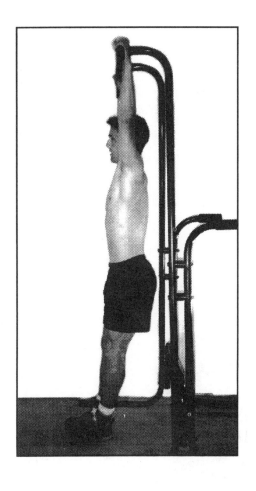

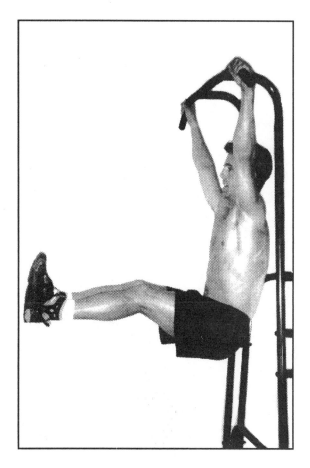

Figure 1

Hang from your pull-up bar with a firm grip...

Figure 2

- Raise your feet up toward your head, as high as you can, while keeping your upper body as stable as possible.

- **Do not drop your legs quickly. To avoid back injury, lower your legs slowly.**

- Do not rock, instead, isolate your abs and allow them to pull your legs up.

42. Floor Knee-Up

If you do not have a pull-up bar, you can get the same effect by following the demonstration below.

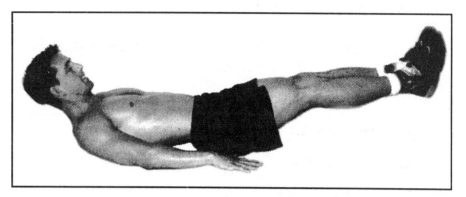

Figure 1

- Lay on your back.
- Raise your heels 6" off the ground.

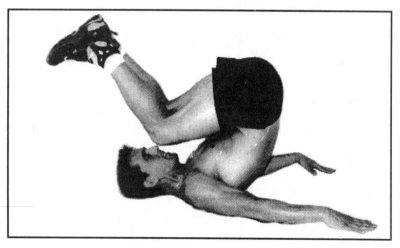

Figure 2

- Now bring your knees to your chest, as shown above.
- To prevent injury, do not go past the vertical position when curling your legs to your chest.
- This exercise is similar to the Hanging Knee-Up [#41], but the key to this exercise is that when you lower your legs, do not let your feet touch the ground.
- Only when the set is over may you lower your feet to the ground. **No cheating!**

III. Lower Body Workout

Beginner

To Start: Perform this exercise program Monday, Wednesday and Friday—
              for four weeks.

Progress: After four weeks, advance to five times a week.

Cobra Stretch: See page 31.

Exercise	Repetitions	
1. Regular Sit-Up	10	
2. Half Sit-Up	10	
3. Hand to Toe	10	
4. Cobra Stretch	**3**	
5. Crunch	10	
6. Side Sit-Up (Each side)	5	
7. Oblique (Each side)	5	
8. Cobra Stretch	**3**	
9. Flutter Kick	4	[Count 10]
10. Leg Raise	10	
11. Cutting Edge	4	[Count 10]
12 Cobra Stretch	**3**	
13. Knee Bend	10	
14. Helen Keller	10	
15. Hanging Knee-Up (2 Sets)	5	
16. Cobra Stretch	**3**	
17. Hanging Leg-Up	10	
18. Floor Knee-Up	10	
19. Trunk Extensions	5	

III. Lower Body Workout

Intermediate

To Start: Perform this exercise program Monday, Wednesday and Friday—
              for four weeks.

Progress: After four weeks, advance to five times a week.

Cobra Stretch: See page 31.

Exercise		Repetitions	
1.	Regular Sit-Up	30	
2.	Half Sit-Up	30	
3.	Hand to Toe	30	
4.	**Cobra Stretch**	**3**	
5.	Crunch	30	
6.	Side Sit-Up (Each side)	30	
7.	Oblique (Each side)	30	
8.	**Cobra Stretch**	**3**	
9.	Flutter Kick	4	[Count 10]
10.	Leg Raise	30	
11.	Cutting Edge	4	[Count 10]
12.	**Cobra Stretch**	**3**	
13.	Knee Bend	30	
14.	Helen Keller	30	
15.	Hanging Knee-Up (2 Sets)	15	
16	**Cobra Stretch**	**3**	
17.	Hanging Leg-Up (2 Sets)	10	
18.	Floor Knee-Up	30	
19.	Trunk Extensions	10	

III. Lower Body Workout

Advanced

- You will now be doing two sets of each exercise.
- Complete a full cycle (one set) before moving on to the second cycle.
- Perform the following exercise program five times a week.
- Cobra Stretch: See page 31.

Exercise	Repetitions
1. Regular Sit-Up	2 x 35
2. Half Sit-Up	2 x 35
3. Hand to Toe	2 x 35
4. Cobra Stretch	**3**
5. Crunch	2 x 35
6. Side Sit-Up (Each side)	2 x 35
7. Oblique (Each side)	2 x 35
8. Cobra Stretch	**3**
9. Flutter Kick	2 x 4 Count 35
10. Leg Raise	2 x 35
11. Cutting Edge	2 x 4 Count 35
12. Cobra Stretch	**3**
13. Knee Bend	2 x 35
11. Helen Keller	2 x 35
12. Hanging Knee-Up (2 Sets)	2 x 35
13. Cobra Stretch	**3**
14. Hanging Leg-Up (2 Sets)	2 x 35
15. Floor Knee-Up	2 x 35
16. Trunk Extensions	10

IV.   Running

IV.   Running

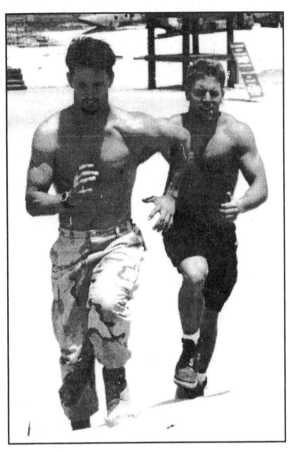

Running can sometimes be a controversial subject. Some may live and breathe by running, and others may have nothing good to say about it. Personally, I do not have a Ph.D in physiology or science, but running has been a major part of my life and career, and I can tell you that you can receive great joy from it. Not just for the physical benefits, but the peace of mind that you enter while you run can be very relaxing.

As far as SEALs and BUD/S go, running is practically a daily ritual. Men have been made and men have been broken by excruciating runs during SEAL training. SEAL teams run as a team three times a week and most everyone runs on their own during the other days of the week. As a Navy SEAL, I have fond memories and also bitter memories of running during my training at BUD/S.

I've always enjoyed heading out to an empty, tourist-free beach and running as the sun sets. I pick a nice, steady pace, and as the sun goes down I feel my worries and concerns leaving along with it. There's nothing quite like it. I love feeling the water splash on my bare feet. What a great way to get away from it all and relieve some tension. Nearly every Friday evening I would jog the beaches of beautiful San Diego, clearing my mind and putting me into a great mood as I thought about picking up my girfriend, Cristina, for a night of dancing.

Then there are the bitter memories of running during SEAL training. Our physical training leader, Instructor Jared, had just PT'd (exercised) us to death and was standing up front, ready to take us out for a run. After a grueling session, this guy hadn't even broken a sweat!

Whenever Instructor Jared ran us, we knew it was going to be a "death march!" He may not of been the fastest instructor at BUD/S, but his stamina was unbelievable. I would rather run behind the fastest instructor on a long road run, than have to run behind an instructor who runs us up and down sand burms and through soft sand. Sure enough—that's where Instructor Jared would take us. He would never break stride, not even in the softest sand!

Instructor Jared also usually had the biggest "Goon Squad." The Goon Squad is the unfortunate group of runners who fall behind the leader, usually lagging about 30 to 60 yards back (varying on each instructor's current mood). Instructor Jared would put us through grueling runs, hoping to create a big Goon Squad. The Goon Squad is given a warning to catch up—or else. Then, if they don't catch up, they get hammered with more and more P.T. It was not uncommon to see someone pass out or drop down from fatigue, just trying to keep up with the team. This is how I learned to dig deep down inside myself to accomplish things I never knew I was capable of doing.

If you have never included running in your training program, or if perhaps you have not been running for a long time, I recommend starting out very slow and easy, to prevent shin splints and stress fractures. I also recommend running at the end of your workout, since your muscles

> *If you have never included running in your training program. or if perhaps you have not been running for a long ime, I recommend starting out very slow and easy, to prevent shin splints and stress fractures.*

will be good and warm, even if they are a little tired from exercising. This is the best time for growth—and you will not have to run a long distance to get the same effect.

Try to add variety to your running, to spice it up a little. Like anything done over and over again, running can become very boring and dull if done on the same course, and in the same manner. I recommend running long distances on Monday, Wednesday and Friday. On Tuesday and Thursday, go to a nearby track and do wind sprints.[1] Another great way to work on speed, strength and stamina is by doing sprints *uphill*. This is an awesome workout! I know it is—because I had to do hundreds of sprints up soft sand burms during BUD/S training. The goal is to work on both speed and endurance. By following this program, you will achieve both.

---

[1] A "wind sprint" is short distance running, going back and forth from one designated spot to another.

I realize that most people dislike sprints, but by ordering this workout program you have proven that you are not just *anyone*.   You are someone who's ready to push their body to its maximum limit to achieve a rock-hard body.

> *"...by ordering this workout program you have proven that you are not just anyone. You are someone who's ready to push their body to its maximum limit to achieve a rock-hard body."*

By doing sprints, you train the muscle fibers in your legs to react quickly. This will generate greater development and improve your body's speed in "short burst" situations. Your legs are made up of fast twitch fibers and slow twitch fibers. By running long distances, you work the slow twitch fibers. Include wind sprints once a week to work the fast twitch fibers. Sprints will improve the over-all development of your legs.

Be creative and make your running enjoyable. Once your running or sprint session is finished, spend a little time stretching out. I'm not talking about a marathon stretch session—just a couple of minutes of stretching will help you prevent injuries and improve your flexibility.

IV. Running Program

Beginner

First Week

Monday	1 mile
Tuesday	1/2 mile or 900 yards jogging first 200 yards, then sprinting for 100 yards and so on, up to 900 yards.
Wednesday	1 mile
Thursday	Sprint 100 yards and jog 100 yards, up to 100 yards.
Friday	1 mile

Second Week

Monday	1 mile
Tuesday	Stair Sprints (stairs, bleachers, hills) Five minutes total time*
Wednesday	1 mile
Thursday	1/2 mile or 900 yards
Friday	1 1/2 mile

* Pick a 25 foot section of stairs to sprint up—then jog down.   You want to continually push yourself. *No walking in this exercise!*

• Each person's fitness level varies, so take it slow to find your limitation. If you have never sprinted up stairs before, you'll find out that it is tougher than it looks.

• Do not attempt the Advanced level straight out of the gate. Your stamina will increase, but you must work toward it in moderation. You will increase your distance 1/2 mile every two weeks.

IV. Running Program

Intermediate

First Week

Monday	3 miles
Tuesday	1 mile. Jog 300 yards. Sprint 150 yards, up to 1800 yards.
Wednesday	3 miles
Thursday	Jog 100 yards. Sprint 100 yards, up to 1800 yards.
Friday	3 miles

Second Week

Monday	3 mile
Tuesday	Stair Sprints, ten minutes total. 50 feet in length.
Wednesday	3 miles
Thursday	1 mile. Jog 300 yards. Sprint 150 yards, up to 1800 yards.
Friday	3 1/2 miles

IV. Running Program
Advanced

First Week

Monday	4 miles
Tuesday	1 1/2 miles. Jog 300 yards. Sprint 150 yards, up to 2700 yards.
Wednesday	4 miles
Thursday	Jog 100 yards. Sprint 100 yards, up to 2700 yards.
Friday	4 miles

Second Week

Monday	4 mile
Tuesday	Stair Sprints, fifteen minutes total, 100 feet in length.
Wednesday	4 miles
Thursday	1 1/2 miles. Jog 300 yards. Sprint 150 yards, up to 2700 yards.
Friday	4 1/2 miles

* Once you have reached the advanced program, your progress does not stop. This program is just the minimum, which means you will continue to increase in increments of 1/2 mile every two weeks, up to six miles. You can stay at this level or continue on.

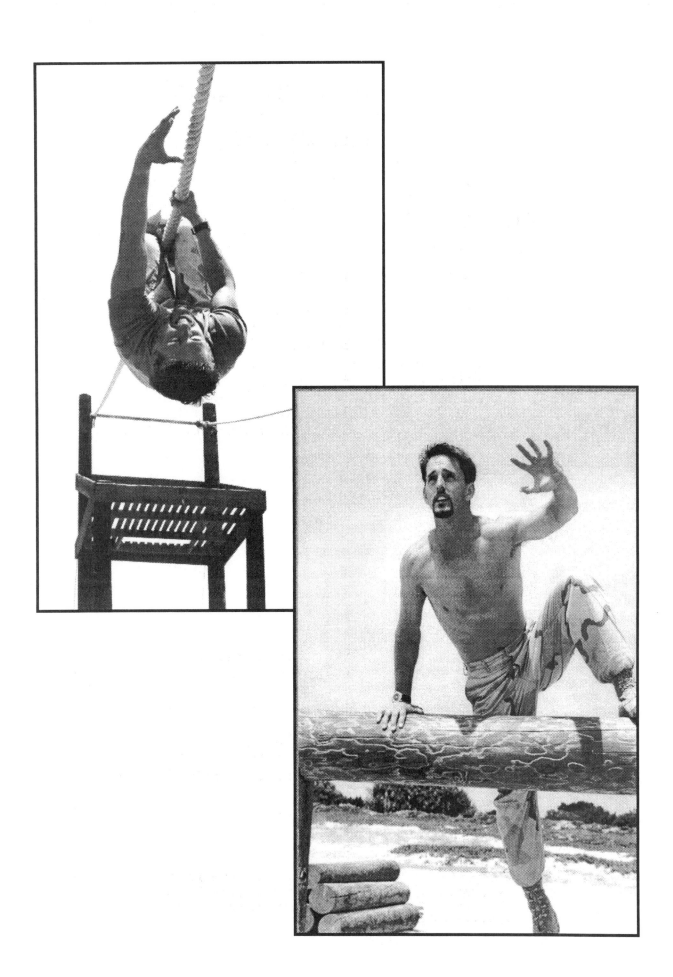

V. Swimming

V.   Swimming

Many people like the physiques of swimmers, with their sleek and hard muscles. It seems as though they have every muscle developed, with no weak areas. Men and women dream of being as toned as swimmers. The thing is, all these aspirations and dreams will remain just that—if you don't jump in and get wet.

Unfortunately, not everyone has access to a swimming pool. If not, just remember the things I'm going to discuss and when you do have access to a pool, use them then. You don't have to have a swimming pool in your backyard. There are pools at club houses, community centers, high schools and at colleges. Somehow, try to find regular access to a pool because swimming is probably the best way to improve your over-all fitness.

" ...swimming is probably the best way to improve your over-all fitness."

Swimming should be broken up into several strokes. During BUD/S training we were taught two strokes: "freestyle" and the "side stroke" [or UDT stroke].

We achieved the best results when we alternated between using fins and going barefoot. I recommend using swimming fins to assist your strokes, and eye goggles to protect your eyes from chlorine. These products are available in the Cutting Edge product catalogue [see page 112], or can be purchased at a local sporting goods store. Another useful item for swimming is a flotation device. These products will allow you to jog in the pool with zero stress to the body.

Later on in the program, I will give you an outline to follow for swimming. Just remember that swimming can be one of the most beneficial exercises you can do.   Once again, before you begin any strenuous exercise—remember to stretch.   The upper body stretches will work great for your swimming routine [see pages 16 through 23.

SEALs are like fish in the water, and we are extremely comfortable there. During BUD/S training we swam up to 5,000 yards a day.

It was amazing to see the great shape swimming helped us to achieve.

V. Swimming Program
Beginner

Monday	Freestyle stroke for 600 yards.
Tuesday	Breast stroke for 300 yards.
Wednesday	Freestyle stroke for 600 yards.
Thursday	Side stroke for 600 yards.
Friday	Freestyle stroke for 600 yards.

* Every two weeks increase your distance 100 yards.

V. Swimming Program
Intermediate

Monday	Freestyle stroke for 1200 yards.
Tuesday	Breast stroke for 600 yards.
Wednesday	Freestyle stroke for 1200 yards.
Thursday	Side stroke for 1200 yards.
Friday	Freestyle stroke for 1200 yards.

- Every two weeks increase your distance 100 yards.

V. Swimming Program
Advanced

Monday	Freestyle stroke for 1800 yards.
Tuesday	Breast stroke for 900 yards.
Wednesday	Freestyle stroke for 1800 yards.
Thursday	Side stroke for 1800 yards.
Friday	Freestyle stroke for 1800 yards.

- Every two weeks increase your distance 100 yards.

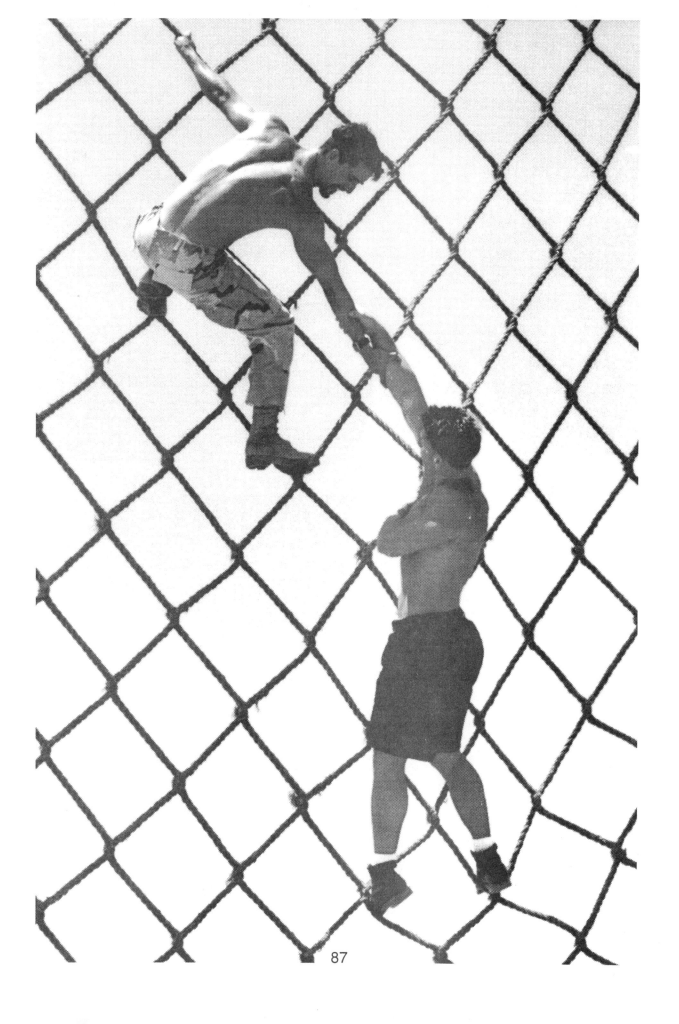

VI. Combined Program

VI. Combined Program

Beginner

First Week

Monday	1 mile run.
Tuesday	Freestyle stroke for 600 yards.
Wednesday	1/2 mile sprint. Jog 300 yards. Sprint 150 yards up to 900 yards.
Thursday	Freestyle stroke for 400 yards. Breast stroke for 200 yards.
Friday	1 mile run.

Second Week

Monday	1 mile run.
Tuesday	Freestyle stroke for 600 yards.
Wednesday	Stair Sprints, 25 feet, five minutes.
Thursday	Freestyle stroke for 400 yards. Side stroke for 200 yards.
Friday	1 1/2 mile run.

VI. Combined Program
Intermediate

First Week

Monday	3 mile run.
Tuesday	Freestyle stroke for 1200 yards.
Wednesday	1 mile sprint. Jog 300 yards. Sprint 150 yards up to 1800 yards.
Thursday	Freestyle stroke for 800 yards. Breast stroke for 400 yards.
Friday	3 mile run.

Second Week

Monday	3 mile run.
Tuesday	Freestyle stroke for 1200 yards.
Wednesday	Stair Sprints, 50 feet, ten minutes.
Thursday	Freestyle stroke for 800 yards. Side stroke for 400 yards.
Friday	3 1/2 mile run.

VI. Combined Program
Advanced

First Week

Monday	4 mile run.
Tuesday	Freestyle stroke for 1800 yards.
Wednesday	1 1/2 mile sprint. Jog 300 yards. Sprint 150 yards up to 2700 yards.
Thursday	Freestyle stroke for 1200 yards. Breast stroke for 600 yards.
Friday	4 mile run.

Second Week

Monday	4 mile run.
Tuesday	Freestyle stroke for 1800 yards.
Wednesday	Stair Sprints, 100 feet, fifteen minutes.
Thursday	Freestyle stroke for 1200 yards. Side stroke for 600 yards.
Friday	4 1/2 mile run.

VII. Cool Down

VII. Cool Down

Cooling down is an important step in the recovery of your muscles. Any time you engage in strenuous exercise it is necessary to carefully stretch out your muscles to prevent pulls and intense soreness. You are not going to avoid soreness—you are going to be sore for about the first two weeks. But don't worry, your body will adjust to your new schedule. **Soreness means growth.** There is a difference between soreness and *pain*. If your body feels sharp pain you may be over exerting yourself, and you could be pulling or tearing a muscle. Take it easy and let your muscles recover. If you do pull a muscle, then stop training and begin stretching carefully and slowly. Do this several times a day for the next couple of days until the pain goes away. To prevent injuries, make sure you're stretching out properly before and after your workout. If you choose to workout every other day, then on your off days, stretch out in the mornings for 10 minutes.

When cooling down from running, do not go straight to a bench and sit down. Even though you're tired–that is the worst thing you can do because your muscles are going to tighten up. Muscles need to be slowly cooled down, rather than completely shut down. As tired as you may be, stay up and walk around slowly for at least five minutes. This will slowly cool your muscles down and prepare them for shut down.

" ... here you have a workout program successfully used by the finest combat forces in the world—and all you have to do is follow the instructions ."

When cooling down after swimming, use the same stretches you used before your workout. There is nothing wrong with adding to these stretches. I have included only the basic stretches and exercises. So if you learn something new from someone else, incorporte it into this workout. That's the simplicity of this program. Just make sure you're using the proper form. This program will give you a solid foundation to build upon, and grow along with you.

This program works, there's no doubt about it. I've seen it work miracles, and I know it works because it worked for me. With anything in life, you'll get out of it what you put into it. Do not expect to achieve miraculous results working out for only 10 minutes, once a week. **It takes times and dedication.** You ordered this book expecting a complete body workout. Well—here you have a workout program successfully used by the finest combat forces in the world— and all you have to do is follow the instructions.

This this is a time-tested, proven method to physical fitness perfection! And now it is in your hands. You can put it on your bookshelf or throw it in your closet, and stay at your current fitness level. Or you can tear into this book and get into the best shape of your life.

It worked for me—and it **will** work for you!

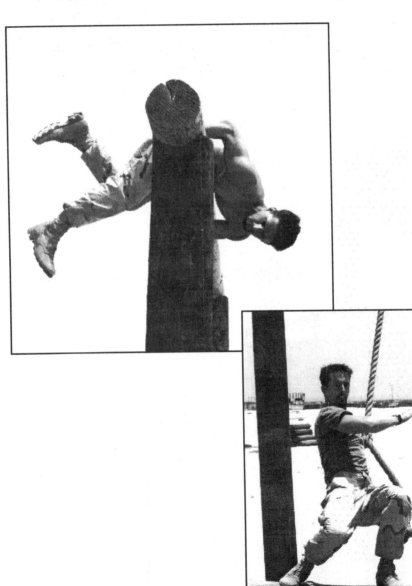

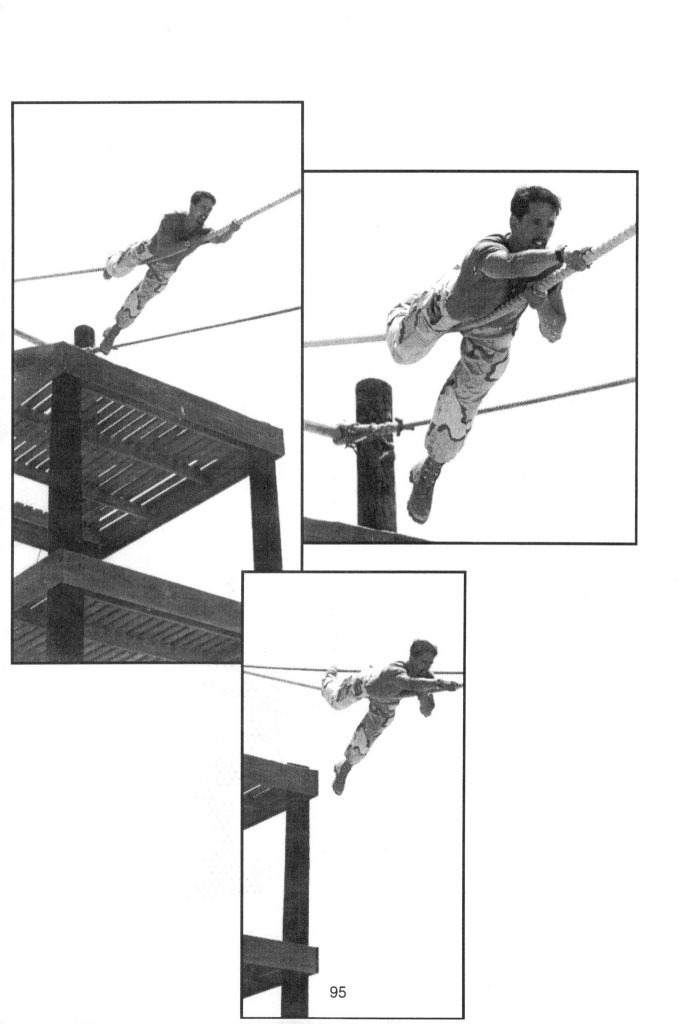

VIII. Diet & Nutrition

VIII.   Diet & Nutrition

by Dr. Christine DuPraw

Professor of Nutrition
MESA COLLEGE
San Diego, California

What To Eat

Since Carbohydrates are the primary fuel for the working muscle, the diet should be rich in starches such as pasta, bread, cereals, beans, fruits and vegetables. A good variety of foods will ensure getting enough vitamins and minerals. The USDA's Food Guide Pyramid is a useful guide to know how many servings to eat each day. Note that the foundation of the diet is carbohydrate based.

The number of servings you select should depend on your activity level and size. If you choose the maximum servings from each food group you would consume about 2800 calories. The more active you are, the more calories you will need to maintain your weight. Most people who exercise benefit from a high carbohydrate, low fat diet.[1] This diet would provide about 60-70% of the calories coming from carbohydrate, 15% from protein and 15-25% from fat. Saturated animal fats like butter should be minimized and when possible, replaced with plant oils, such as canola, olive or peanut.

Concern about vitamins and minerals should be taken if the person does not eat a variety of food or drops below 1500 calories a day. With greater physical activity, most people eat more and as long as the food is wholesome, vitamin and mineral needs will be met. In general, large doses of individual vitamins and minerals have not been shown to help an already well-nourished athlete. A person wishing to take a supplement should choose one that offers 100-200% of the U.S. RDA[2] of vitamins and minerals.

For individuals engaged in intense exercise, a greater intake of fruits and vegetables is advised. These foods help provide antioxidant nutrients (e.g. vitamin C, beta-carotene) which may protect the body from a potential increase of harmful "free radical" chemicals. By purchasing a food composition guide or nutritional analysis software, you would be able to figure your calorie and nutrient intake. Remember that supplements will not take the place of a healthy diet. If you feel you need more individualized nutrition counseling, please contact SCAN[3] (Sports and Cardiovascular Nutritionalists).

---

[1] Low fat diet: It is recommended to increase vitamin E intake to 200 mg.

[2] United States Department of Agriculture, Recommended Daily Allowance

[3] SCAN - Sports Nutrition Institute: Telephone: (303) 779-1950

For most people, a one pound muscle gain per week is a reasonable goal to set. At this time it is not known how many calories are needed to make one pound of muscle tissue, nor in what form these calories should be in. An estimate is that you would need to eat 400-500 extra calories a day to gain one pound of muscle each week. However, if you have a fast metabolism or are also participating in intense aerobic activity, you may require more calories. Be careful of caffeine and smoking—both increase metabolism.

The increase in calories should come primarily from carbohydrates with a small increase in protein and fat. One pound of muscle is about 22% (100 grams) protein, 70% water and 7% fat. Therefore, to gain one pound of muscle in a week, 14 grams of additional protein per day would need to be eaten. This can easily be met by adding 2 cups of milk, 2 ounces of meat, fish or poultry, or 2 ounces of cheese. Protein powders and amino acid supplements are not necessary and can be expensive. Research studies have suggested that only 7 - 28 grams of protein per day can be retained for muscle growth.

For athletes, another way to estimate how much protein you need is to multiply your weight in kilograms (lbs. divided by 2.2 = kilograms) by 1.5 - 1.75 grams of protein. For example, a 150 lb. person would weigh 68 kg. and should consume a maximum of 120 grams of protein each day. A 3 ounce portion of meat, fish or chicken provides about 21 grams of protein, and a cup of milk or yogurt supplies about 9 grams. Protein is easy to come by, but expensive amounts are not related to greater muscle development.

The remaining calories should come from whole grain breads, cereals, pastas and vegetables. Avoid using saturated animal fats. Instead, substitute plant oils, such as canola, olive and avocado. It is very difficult for some people to gain weight unless they consume about 30% of their daily calories from fat. It should be emphasized that the source of this fat should come from plants rather than animals, e.g. a peanut butter sandwich (avoid hydrogenated[4] peanut butter) on whole wheat bread would make a healthy, high energy snack. For those who get tired of always having to fix food, "liquid meals" [such as Ensure and other "weight gain" supplements] come in handy. A single serving can provide an additional 400 calories in a quick, easy to swallow drink.

---

[4] Hydrogenation refers to the process of converting plant oil to a creamy consistency (such as margarine or Crisco), which affects the texture and appearance of food products. Hydrogenated foods contain saturated fat, which raises cholesterol.

To Lose Weight

One pound of fat contains 3500 calories. By creating a daily deficit of 500 calories you can lose one pound of fat per week. A loss of one to two pounds per week is considered a safe weight loss. The only way to lose the fat and keep it off is to commit to eating a low (about 20%) fat diet and increasing your activity. Many people are successful in losing weight by simply looking at where the fat is in their diet and substituting low or non-fat food. Fat provides over twice as many calories as carbohydrates and protein. Caution must be taken not to overeat non-fat or low fat foods. Many non-fat baked products add extra sugar so they are still a good source of calories.

Excessive calories from carbohydrate, protein or fat will cause weight gain if not burned in physical activity. Exercise helps in weight loss, not only by burning more calories, but by increasing metabolism due to increases in lean body mass. The more muscle tissue developed, the more calories you will burn, even while relaxing. Exercise increases self-esteem which reinforces healthy diet changes. Focus on what you can do, rather than what you can eat. Here are some tips that help:

- Eat breakfast.
- Drink lots of water.
- Do not eat while watching television.
- Do not eat fast.

To Gain Weight

A person may be underweight for a variety of reasons, e.g., medical, emotional, or from inheriting a fast metabolism. The goal in gaining weight is to gain muscle, not fat. Successful weight gains are achieved by:

- Eating more frequently.
- Getting adequate sleep and rest.
- Participating in a progressive resistance training program.

Progressive weight training with heavier weights causes the greatest stimulus to muscle development and the caloric burn is relatively little compared to more active aerobic exercise. A medical check-up should be obtained before starting a heavy weight lifting program.

The Cutting Edge
Food Guide Pyramid
A Guide to Daily Food Choices

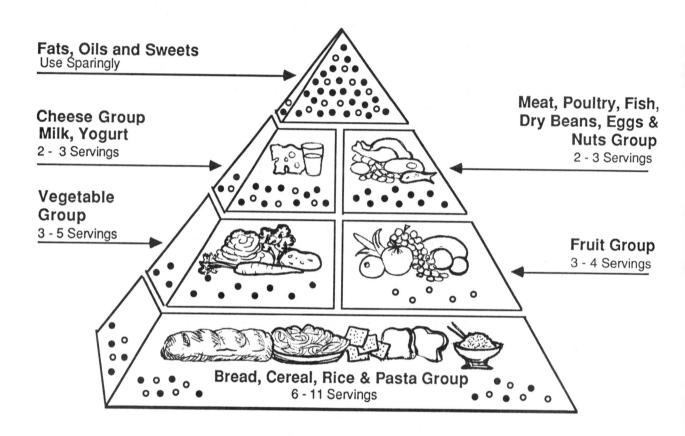

Fats, Oils and Sweets
Use Sparingly

Cheese Group
Milk, Yogurt
2 - 3 Servings

Vegetable
Group
3 - 5 Servings

Meat, Poultry, Fish,
Dry Beans, Eggs &
Nuts Group
2 - 3 Servings

Fruit Group
3 - 4 Servings

Bread, Cereal, Rice & Pasta Group
6 - 11 Servings

Symbol Key

● **Fat**   [Naturally occurring and added]

○ **Sugars**   [Added]

These symbols show that fats and added sugars come
mostly from fats, oils, and sweets, but can be part of
[or added to] foods from the other food groups as well.

Nutrition Guide

Pyramid Food Group	Serving Size
Milk, Yogurt, Cheese	1 Cup of milk or yogurt. 1 1/2 ounces natural cheese. 2 ounces of processed cheese.
Meat, Poultry, Fish, Dry Beans, Eggs & Nuts	2 - 3 ounces of cooked, lean meat, poultry or fish. 1/2 cup of cooked dry beans. 1 egg. 2 tablespoons peanut butter.
Bread, Cereal, Rice and Pasta	1 slice of bread. 1 ounce of ready-to-eat cereal. 1/2 cup of cooked cereal, rice or pasta.
Vegetables	1 cup of raw, leafy vegetables. 1/2 cup of other vegetables, cooked or chopped raw. 3/4 cup vegetable juice.
Fruit	1 medium apple, banana, or orange. 1/2 cup of chopped, cooked or canned fruit. 3/4 cup of fruit juice.
Fats, Oils, Sweets (Not an official food group)	No serving size.

IX.   Progress Charts

IX. Progress Charts

In the next three pages I have included three charts, which I strongly urge you to use to monitor your progress. They will keep you motivated because as you see yourself improving, you will want to continue this program with even more desire.

The first step in using these charts is to record the date you started the program, your starting weight, and the date each chart is finished. As you progress, continue to record your weight.

The second step is to do the workouts and record your starting ability for each exercise in the "starting ability" column. In a couple of months you are going to be amazed at how many repetitions you will be able to achieve.

The next step is to list your goals. As I said before... *a goal not written is only a dream.* Listing your goals will keep you on track for success and hold you accountable for your performance. The "goal" I am referring to is the number of repetitions you want to be able to perform for each individual exercise at that stage of the program. List your goal for the completion of the second week. Then list your long term goal in the goal column on the far right. This will be a little bit more difficult to accurately predict, since it is eight weeks away.

"Do not get discouraged if your measurements and weight stay the same for a couple of months. Your body is adjusting to its new routine."

Don't get discouraged! By the time you reach the second chart, you should be able to reach your long term goal easier because you will be able to better predict your performance. Once you complete the second week, list your goal for the end of the fourth week. Once you complete the fourth week, list your goal for the end of the sixth week. Continue on in this manner. Your short term goals are going to be a bit more realistic than your long term ones. This is not a problem. As long as you progress steadily and improve your physical fitness, you have nothing to fear.

Other important goals for you to set are your desired weight and measurements. Measure the size of your waist, chest, arms, legs and neck. Before you start the program, get a measuring tape and record the starting date and your measurements. Get a friend to help you measure yourself. Record your measurements every month thereafter, on the same day of the month. For instance, if you recorded your weight and measurements on October 8, then weigh and measure yourself again on November 8, and on the 8th day of every month thereafter. Write everything down so you can see yourself progressing on paper.

Do not get discouraged if your measurements and weight stay the same for a couple of months. Your body is adjusting to its new routine. Also, since muscle weighs more than fat, you may remain the same weight, but your waist size should go down. This is because your muscles are going to grow due to the intensity of the upper body program. As your muscles grow, you are going to gain weight. At the same time, running and swimming will burn fat. So, you may remain the same weight for a few months. Again, *don't get discouraged.* Be happy that you are burning off excess fat—and gaining hard-earned muscle.

When you are finished with the first three charts, take the Master Chart and photocopy it. The blank Master Chart will enable you to make as many charts as you need to monitor your physical progress.

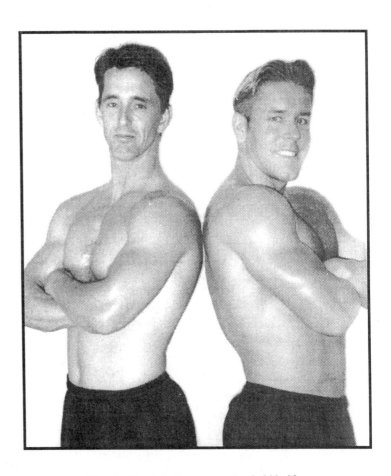

Mark De Lisle   R. J. Wolf

Cutting Edge
Progress Record

Before...

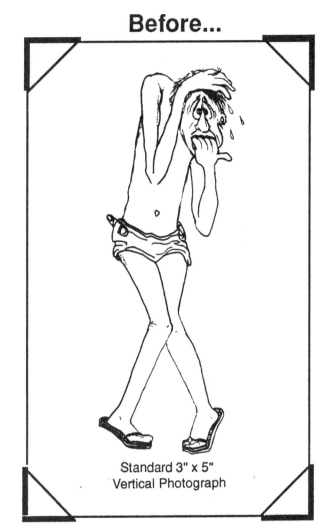

Standard 3" x 5"
Vertical Photograph

After !

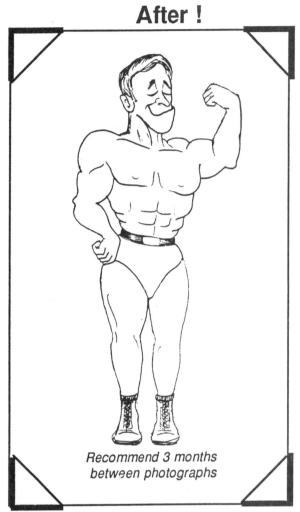

Recommend 3 months
between photographs

MEASUREMENTS

		Before...	3 Months	6 Months	9 Months	After!
1.	DATE					
2.	Weight					
3.	Neck					
4.	Chest					
5.	Bicep					
6.	Tricep					
7.	Waist					
8.	Hips (Female)					
9.	Thigh					
10.	Calf					

Navy SEAL Exercises Weekly Workout Chart
Your Cutting Edge Roadmap to a Chiseled Body!

Exercise	STARTING ABILITY	Week # ___		Week # ___		Week # ___		Week # ___		ENDING GOAL
		GOAL	Accom-plished	GOAL	Accom-plished	GOAL	Accom-plished	GOAL	Accom-plished	
Pull-Ups										
Regular										
Reverse										
Close-Grip										
Behind the Neck										
Commando										
Bar Dips										
Regular										
Push-Ups										
Regular										
Tricep										
Dive Bomber										
Wide Angle										
Sit-Ups										
Regular										
Half Sit-Up										
Hand-to-Toe										
Crunch										
Oblique										
Side Sit-Up										
Flutter Kick										
Leg Raise										
Cutting Edge										
Knee Bend										
Helen Keller										
Knee-Up										
Leg-Up										
Floor Knee-Up										

Navy SEAL Exercises Weekly Workout Chart
Your Cutting Edge Roadmap to a Chiseled Body!

Exercise	STARTING ABILITY	Week # ___		Week # ___		Week # ___		Week # ___		ENDING GOAL
		GOAL	Accomplished	GOAL	Accomplished	GOAL	Accomplished	GOAL	Accomplished	
Pull-Ups										
Regular										
Reverse										
Close-Grip										
Behind the Neck										
Commando										
Bar Dips										
Regular										
Push-Ups										
Regular										
Tricep										
Dive Bomber										
Wide Angle										
Sit-Ups										
Regular										
Half Sit-Up										
Hand-to-Toe										
Crunch										
Oblique										
Side Sit-Up										
Flutter Kick										
Leg Raise										
Cutting Edge										
Knee Bend										
Helen Keller										
Knee-Up										
Leg-Up										
Floor Knee-Up										

MASTER - Workout Chart

Exercise	STARTING ABILITY	Week #		Week #		Week #		Week #		ENDING GOAL
		GOAL	Accomplished	GOAL	Accomplished	GOAL	Accomplished	GOAL	Accomplished	
Pull-Ups										
Regular										
Reverse										
Close-Grip										
Behind the Neck										
Commando										
Bar Dips										
Regular										
Push-Ups										
Regular										
Tricep										
Dive Bomber										
Wide Angle										
Sit-Ups										
Regular										
Half Sit-Up										
Hand-to-Toe										
Crunch										
Oblique										
Side Sit-Up										
Flutter Kick										
Leg Raise										
Cutting Edge										
Knee Bend										
Helen Keller										
Knee-Up										
Leg-Up										
Floor Knee-Up										

Personal Notes

X. Cutting Edge Fitness

X. Cutting Edge Fitness

"Open Door"

We have an "open-door" policy at Cutting Edge Fitness. If you have any questions, suggestions or comments—we encourage you to call or write:

Cutting Edge Fitness
4901 Morena Boulevard
Suite 127
San Diego, California 92117

1 (800) 281-SEAL (7325)

Cutting Edge Products

You are invited to sample the Cutting Edge clothing, product and supplement line. It is full of exciting sports apparel, equipment to assist you with the Navy SEAL exercise manual, and proven nutritional supplements to help your growth nd recovery rates.

To receive a complimentary copy of our product brochure, or to order additional copies of *Navy SEAL Exercises: Cutting Edge Total Body Workout,* Please call or write:

Cutting Edge Fitness
4901 Morena Boulevard
Suite 127
San Diego, California 92117

1 (800) 281-SEAL (7325)

Fitness Demonstrations

Cutting Edge staff members are also available for company or fitness center demonstrations. If you represent a fitness center or gym, and would like your staff trained in this program, please call or write:

Cutting Edge Fitness
4901 Morena Boulevard
Suite 127
San Diego, California 92117

1 (800) 281-SEAL (7325)

We are always available to give you support and assistance with any aspect of your fitness training, so please do not hesitate to request our help.

In the interim, I truly hope that you get as much out of this program as I have.

Good luck!

I know you can do it!

— Mark De Lisle

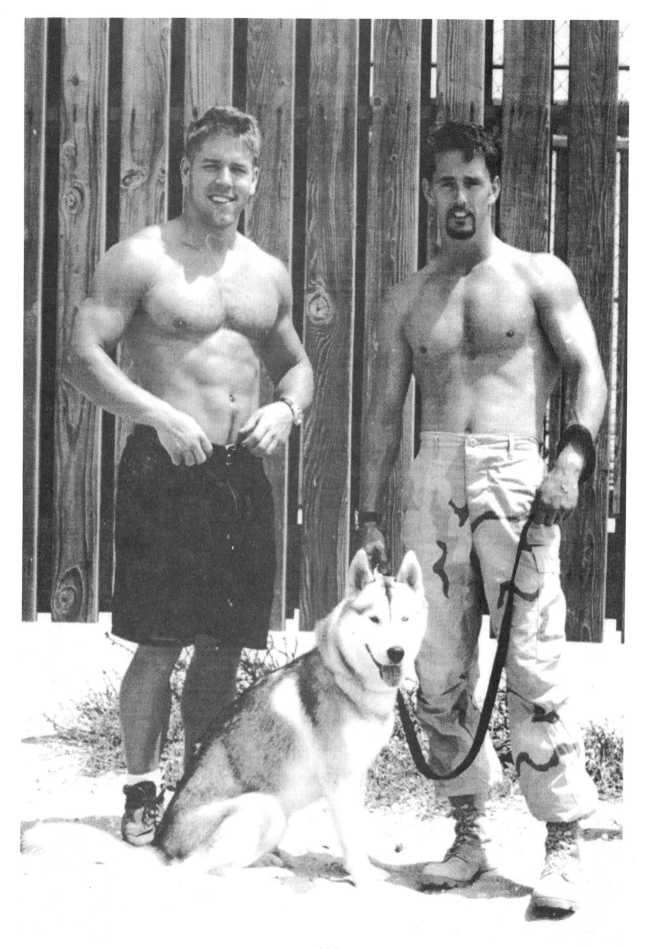